# Using Occupational Therapy Theory in Practice

Edited by

**Gail Boniface** PhD, MSc, DipCOT
*Cardiff University*

**Alison Seymour** MSc, BSc, DipCOT
*Cardiff University*

Foreword by M. Clare Taylor

D1246308

**(W)WILEY-BLACKWELL**

A John Wiley & Sons, Ltd., Publication

*Library of Congress Cataloging-in-Publication Data*
Using occupational therapy theory in practice / edited by Gail Boniface, Alison Seymour.
    p. ; cm.
 Includes bibliographical references and index.
 ISBN 978-1-4443-3317-6 (pbk. : alk. paper)
 I. Boniface, Gail.  II. Seymour, Alison.
 [DNLM:  1. Occupational Therapy.  2. Models, Theoretical. WB 555]
 LC classification not assigned
 615.8′515–dc23

                                                            2011034240

A catalogue record for this book is available from the British Library.

Set in 10/12.5pt Times by Aptara® Inc., New Delhi, India
Printed and bound in Malaysia by Vivar Printing Sdn Bhd

1   2012

# Contents

# Contributor biographies

## Editors

### Gail Boniface
*PhD, MSc in Medical Education, DipCOT, Cert Ed, Certificate in Supervisory Management*
Gail has worked in occupational therapy education for 23 years and is currently working in the School of Health Care Studies Cardiff University as an occupational therapy programme lead. She has a long-standing interest in the use of occupational therapy theory in practice and has been very much involved in providing courses on the use of models of occupational therapy and supporting practitioners in their use.

### Alison Seymour
*MSc, Postgraduate Certificate in University Teaching and Learning, FHEA, BSc, DipCOT*
Alison has worked in occupational therapy education for 7 years and is currently working in the School of Health Care Studies at Cardiff University. Previous to this, she worked for 19 years in a variety of mental health services including forensic, child and adolescent mental health, community mental health and eating disorder services. She has used a range of occupational therapy models of practice within these settings.

## Contributors

**Andreja Bartolac** qualified in physiotherapy, occupational therapy and psychology. Andreja has been working as a teacher at the Occupational Therapy Department of University of Applied Health Studies in Zagreb, Croatia, since 2001. Her professional interests are in the field of occupational therapy assessment, ergonomics and occupational science. For more than 10 years, she has actively participated in all major events associated with development of the occupational therapy profession in Croatia, through the work in the main board of national association of occupational therapists, establishment of Croatian Chamber of Health Professionals and curriculum development.

**Sarah Cook** (BSc in occupational therapy) is a Clinical Specialist Head of Occupational therapy in the Acute and Crisis Services at South London and Maudsley NHS Trust. She has worked in a variety of NHS trusts across South Wales and London after completing her qualification in 1999. Most of her experience has been in Acute in-patient and Crisis Services, Forensic settings and Assertive Outreach Teams. She is passionate about the use of MOHO in practice and regularly provides workshops on various aspects of the model. She is a visiting lecturer at South Bank University.

**Tamsin Fedden** (DipCOT, PGCert HE, MSc) has worked as an occupational therapist for 28 years. She has worked in Mental Health, Learning Disability, Physical Health and Social Care settings with adults and children and has been employed as a senior lecturer at the University of the West of England. Tamsin is particularly interested in the links between theory and practice and in practitioners' continuing development. She is a member of the Gloucestershire CMOP (Canadian Model of Occupational Performance) steering group.

**Della Fish** (MA, MEd, PhD, Dip Ed, FAcadMed) taught in schools and then in university teacher education for 24 years before becoming an educational consultant in health care education. Her interests are in curriculum design and development and in teaching and learning in the clinical setting. She has worked for The College of Occupational Therapy as an adviser and as their representative in various validation processes, for the Acupuncture Accreditation Board, transitioning private colleges into universities and for The Royal College of Surgeons, helping them to design their first formal curriculum for surgery. She holds chairs in Swansea University, Chester University and Charles Sturt University in Sydney.

**Heather Hurst** (DipCOT, MSc in occupational therapy) has worked in a variety of health and social care settings over the past 20 years. Currently, she is Head Occupational Therapist to a team who provide occupational therapy services for two community hospitals and is studying for a Professional Doctorate. She is very much interested in developing links between the use of occupational therapy theory and clinical practice. She continues to play an active role in implementing a theoretical model within her organisation and chairs the Gloucestershire CMOP (Canadian Model of Occupational Performance) steering group.

**Louise Ingham** qualified as an occupational therapist in 1985. She specialised in adult mental health and was one of the first group of occupational therapists to become established in community mental health teams. In her current clinical role as an advanced practitioner, she supports occupational therapists in North West Wales to retain and develop their professional occupational focus whilst being core MDT members. She also works as a lecturer practitioner in Bangor University.

**Sharon James** (MPhil, DipCOT, Certificate in Supervisory Management) is currently the deputy head of occupational therapy services for Abertawe Bro Morgannwg University Health Board at Morriston Hospital Swansea. She completed a project on outcome measures, which led to the creation of an occupational therapy professional model-led outcome measure: the MOTOM.

**Lisa John** (MSc, BSc (Hons)) is currently Head Occupational Therapist for Adult Mental Health Service in Swansea (ABMU). She previously worked in, and managed a variety of, mental health settings in England and Wales including, forensic, substance misuse and general mental health. She is currently involved in developing an occupational therapy service to the Prolific and Persistent Offenders Programme with South Wales Probation Service.

**Linda Keelan** (DipCOT) is an occupational therapist who has worked with people accessing mental health services for 27 years. Her clinical role has been mainly within community mental health settings, and also includes in-patient work with adults, older people's mental health and mental health rehabilitation. Her current role is as lead for occupational therapy and other therapies for mental health services in Abertawe Bro Morgannwg University Health Board, which offers extensive local and regional mental health services. Linda has maintained occupation at the core of her practice and incorporates the occupational therapy philosophy within people and service development.

**Karen Lewis** (MSc, DipCOT) is currently the Occupational Therapy Manager for Morriston Hospital, Swansea, which is part of Abertawe Bro Morgannwg University Health Board. She has worked in a diverse range of settings throughout her career including local authority, mental health and latterly specialising in physical settings. Her areas of practice have more recently included palliative care and neurosciences, during which she was instrumental in setting up a Parkinson's disease Assessment and Treatment Centre in Swansea.

**Magdalena Loska** (PhD, MA, BA) currently works as a senior lecturer at The Maria Grzegorzewska Academy of Special Education and is the head of the Occupational Therapy Department there. She is also a special education teacher, specialising in working with people with physical disabilities and has a number of additional neuro-developmental and sensory integration qualifications. She has contributed to a number of books and written articles on the subject of enabling children with disabilities to become more autonomous. She is also engaged in educating teachers on this topic. Her current interests are in assessing levels of autonomy for children with cerebral palsy and identifying barriers to that autonomy.

**Margot Mason** (BSc, Postgraduate Diploma in Occupational Therapy) has worked in Adult Social Care occupational therapy for 16 years and is currently working as a Community Occupational Therapy Manager for NHS Gloucestershire Care Services.

She takes an active interest in service development and the use of evidence-based practice and is a member of the Gloucestershire CMOP steering group.

**Caroline Phelps** qualified in 2002 with a BSc (Hons) in occupational therapy from the school of health professions and rehabilitation sciences in Southampton. Caroline has worked at Gloucestershire Royal Hospital since 2004. Caroline became involved at the very beginning of Gloucestershire's journey in implementing the Canadian Model of Occupational Therapy and was one of the members of the original steering group.

**Ania Pietrzak** (MA in Pedagogical Education, Dip Social Work, Cert Ed, Dip OT) is currently studying for her PhD. Ania has worked in a reformatory school as an occupational therapist. Currently, she works in the Academy of Special Education in Warsaw (Poland) as a lecturer and occupational therapy curriculum co-author. Her field of interest is to develop and adapt Polish occupational therapy to meet the required world standards. She is in the course of creating a new assessment tool for measuring adaptive skills for people with learning disabilities.

**Carly Reagon** (PhD, BSc in occupational therapy) is a lecturer and researcher in the School of Health Care Studies, Cardiff University, Wales. In 2006, she completed a PhD exploring perceptions of evidence-based practice amongst a group of occupational therapists in England.

**Jill Riley** (PhD, MSc in occupational therapy, PG Dip (social science research methods), DipCOT) has been a lecturer in occupational therapy since 1998 and is currently a research coordinator and programme lead for the MSc in occupational therapy in the School of Health Care Studies, Cardiff University. Jill has a special interest in Occupational Science and especially creative occupations and their relationship to health and well-being.

**Gillian Thistlewood** (MSc, DipCOT) currently leads and manages an occupational therapy service over two acute hospitals. After qualifying in 1987 as an occupational therapist, Gillian went on to gain a Master's in Health Sciences (University of London) in 1994. She brings experience, over 23 years, in occupational therapy practice, in a range of clinical and managerial settings. She has worked across teams and inter-professional boundaries and challenges with a range of health care workers. Gillian has an interest in clinical ethics and performance management and is a member of the Gloucestershire CMOP steering group.

**Jane Walker** (MSc, DipCOT) leads and manages an occupational therapy service over a range of health and social care settings, including community hospitals, intermediate care, social care and wheelchair services. She qualified as an occupational therapist in 1984 and gained a Master's in Advanced Occupational Therapy (Plymouth University) in 2008. Her particular interest lies in social care and developing the role of occupational therapists within this practice setting. She is a member of the Gloucestershire CMOP steering group.

**Siân Waygood** (MA in Management and Leadership in Health and Social Care, DipCOT) is currently the Professional Head of Occupational Therapy Services in Gloucestershire. During her time in Gloucestershire, Siân has worked with colleagues and key stakeholders from a range of statutory and voluntary organisations in Gloucestershire on a number of projects to enhance services for Gloucestershire residents including Integration of the Occupational Therapy and Community Equipment Services, introducing Telecare Services and Development of Client-Centred Practice models. Siân is currently a key member of the Gloucestershire CMOP steering group.

# Foreword

The notion of the theory/practice divide and the challenge of applying theory into practice is not new and is something that academics, practitioners and students all struggle with. There are texts about theory but what have been missing are the stories of how to put theory into practice. Whilst the reflectors and theoreticians amongst us might be able to use the strengths of their learning styles to work out how to put theory into their practice, those of us who are pragmatists need to see examples to help us put ideas into practice. Gail Boniface and Alison Seymour and their team of practitioner colleagues have given us the tools and the stories to help cross the theory/practice divide and have combined the 'ivory tower' of the academic world with the 'real life' of practice.

As occupational therapists we see ourselves as practical, pragmatic, hands-on people who get the job done. How many of us when we buy flat-pack furniture skim through the instructions but then just get stuck in trying to build the thing? Practice can seem to be like that, but without the theory and the evidence we cannot articulate our clinical reasoning, as Sarah Cook says in Chapter 12; we might get 'found out', but more importantly we might not be able to give a clear rationale for our role and so we will cease to exist. We need the theories and we need to be able to do as the practitioners in this book have done – we need to be able to tell the story of how theory and models underpin our practice and our actions.

In Chapter 3, Gail Boniface reminds us of the theory of occupational therapy and defines the relevant terms (e.g. model, approach, paradigm) and uses the metaphor of an umbrella to illustrate how theory, models and the professional self must be integrated within practice. Occupational therapists are often accused of being 'jack of all trades' (Drummond 2010) and eclectic. However, the metaphor of the umbrella might help practitioners who feel drawn to an eclectic approach to articulate and justify why eclecticism is appropriate and useful within their practice concept.

One of the key tools for linking theory and practice is evidence-based practice. However, the notion of 'evidence' is contested, as Carly Reagon discusses in Chapter 13. Whilst the use and application of quantitative research evidence, such as RCT and systematic review evidence, is well documented (e.g. Taylor 2007), the integration of the practitioner's experiential knowledge is much more complex and less well articulated. Della Fish, in Chapter 4, explores reflective writing and presents the idea of 'Clinical Reflective Writing' and particularly the idea of the 'rainbow draft' (www.ed4medprac.co.uk/papers.htm) as a potentially valuable tool for articulating the experiential evidence for EBP, as well as supporting evidence for HPC re-registration.

Models and approaches provide us with the toolkit for our occupational therapy practice, irrespective of the practice context or area. They provide us with the tools that underpin clinical reasoning and help us to articulate our practice and to identify the appropriate outcomes, measurements and assessments to utilise. But any tool needs illustration and an instruction manual, with practical examples of how to use it. The seven fascinating and varied chapters that make up Section 2 provide us with just such examples of the challenges and processes of utilising a model within a practice context. Whilst most of the examples are from a relatively narrow geographical area, Chapters 10 and 11 give a broader perspective of occupational therapy within an Eastern European context, providing a fascinating counterpoint to the much more established context of the UK.

Throughout this book, the links between the 'academics' (Gail and Alison) and the practitioners are emphasised. This serves to reiterate the need for academics and practitioners to develop collaborative links, which are not just one way from the university to practice but are two way collaborations building on the skills and strengths of both partners.

I would like to congratulate all of the authors on the development of this text, which I am sure will act as an inspiration for students and practitioners alike in developing their understanding, articulation and use of theory and models within the practice context.

**Dr M. Clare Taylor**
DipCOT, BA (Hons), PGCert, MA (Distinc), PhD
*Lead Therapist*
*School of Health & Social Care*
*Bournemouth University*

## References

Drummond, A. (2010) The Elizabeth Casson Memorial Lecture 2010: 'Jack of all trades and master of none' – the future of occupational therapy? *British Journal of Occupational Therapy* 73(7): 292–299.

Taylor, M.C. (2007) *Evidenced-Based Practice for Occupational Therapists*, 2nd edn. Oxford: Blackwell.

# Chapter 1

# Introduction

*Gail Boniface and Alison Seymour*

In this book (divided into three sections), we invite you to participate in a discussion and debate with us on the use of theory by occupational therapists in relation to today's health and social care settings. A key message throughout the book is our belief that, in order to be able to use theory in practice, it is first necessary to get to grips with that theory and *understand it*. This would appear obvious; but in our experience, we have sometimes found that, for many reasons, when using their theory, practitioners have jumped straight to the use of assessments associated with occupational therapy practice models rather than really understanding the underpinning theory first of all. When this has happened (see Chapters 6, 8 and 12), the model itself has been left behind, a superficial understanding of the use of theory has resulted and the model has eventually been abandoned.

As the preceding paragraph has indicated, this book is both theoretical and practical in nature. It offers definitions of such concepts as professional terminology and occupational therapy professional models, whilst narrating individual practitioners' and services' experiences of using occupational therapy specific theory in practice. More specifically, it aims to:

- consider the nature of professions and professional practice;
- debate the nature of the theory of occupational therapy via the introduction of the concept of models of the profession as an umbrella for practice – this also relates occupational theory to its use in the current evidence-based world of contemporary occupational therapy practice;
- discuss the different ways in which occupational therapists, their support staff and other professionals use theory;
- investigate the practical use of occupational therapy theory and the issues such use raises in health and social care settings from a European perspective;
- investigate the ways in which occupational therapists and their students learn how to use occupational therapy theory in practice;
- relate the use of theory to the nature of the individual therapist as a person; and
- consider the place of reflection as a concept to help the occupational therapist get to grips with their understanding of their own theory base.

*Using Occupational Therapy Theory in Practice*, First Edition. Edited by Gail Boniface and Alison Seymour.
© 2012 Blackwell Publishing Ltd. Published 2012 by Blackwell Publishing Ltd.

## The nature of professions and professional practice

In Chapter 2, a critical lens is offered through which we can begin to reconceptualise both professional practice and identity. We are invited to do this, by reconsidering what it is that makes a professional, a distinct professional working within the organisation, rather than an organisational worker. In the same chapter, we are asked to consider the difference between behaving professionally and being a member of a profession, with loyalty to our professional theories as well as to our employing organisations being viewed as holding equal importance. Here (and in Chapter 5), we are asked to consider what *type* of occupational therapist we are and relate this to our use of our own personality and our moral stance on our practice. In both chapters, we are asked to determine what we feel *counts* as professional practice.

## The theory of occupational therapy and its place in an evidence-based practice world

Chapter 3 offers us an overview of the current models of occupational therapy and puts these in the context of (potentially contentious) definitions of terms associated with professional practice, such as paradigm, philosophy, model and approach. Thus, it takes the theory associated with professions by the horns and provides some clear and usable definitions of terms, which are often discussed and described in an interchangeable and consequently confusing manner elsewhere in occupational therapy literature. The chapter, by so doing, discusses the interrelationship between the concepts the terms represent and provides the context for the chapters in Section 2, wherein practitioners narrate their experiences of using occupational therapy professional models in practice. This definition of the interrelationship of the concepts encourages us to view occupational therapy professional models within the analogy of an umbrella. Chapter 3 should be read in conjunction with Chapter 2, which advocates we take a critical, rather than an unthinking, approach to models of our profession and their use in practice. We should also note here that all of the chapters, wherein practitioners describe their journeys in using occupational therapy professional models, demonstrate the extent to which they have obviously been influenced by the theory, but equally, have altered and tweaked it to fit into their specific working environments. Thus, occupational therapy professional models, clearly having begun in practice, continue to be influenced by that practice.

One of the more recent influences on practice has been the rise of the concept of evidence-based practice, and Chapter 13 relates the theory of the profession to the concept of evidence-based practice more overtly, whilst at the same time asks us to consider what it is that we mean by evidence-based practice. Finally, under this heading of the theory of occupational therapy, we draw attention to the discussion of occupational science in Chapter 14, where its historical and contemporary relationship to occupational therapy is investigated.

## Discussion of the different ways in which occupational therapists, their support staff and other professionals use theory

Throughout the book, the models viewed as those of the profession of occupational therapy are discussed as theories that offer a definition of the profession *and* a process through which the clinical reasoning of the occupational therapist can be demonstrated. Therefore, it is our belief that if a theory of occupational therapy is truly a model of the profession, it should be shared with others; however, this should be done by the occupational therapist using it to explain their reasoning rather than giving it away to others to use. Our reasoning behind this is that if we give our professional models away to other professions, they will not have the occupation theory base that occupational therapists have spent some years both developing and learning about, and which is thus central to *our* models for *our* profession. Equally, we feel that the occupational therapy profession needs to think long and hard about how much of its unique occupational theory it puts under the control of its support staff. Chapter 9 deals with these aspects in more depth and also suggests a delegation and allocation framework for use with support staff when the occupational therapy service as a whole uses an occupational therapy professional model (in this instance, the Canadian Model of Occupational Performance (Townsend et al 2002), now CMOP-E (Townsend and Polatajko 2007)).

## Investigation into the practical use of occupational therapy theory and the issues such use raises in health and social care settings from a European perspective

The whole of Section 2 of this book is dedicated to the practical use of occupational therapy professional models in service settings. The narratives of the services and the staff implementing the models have been described by the practitioners in detail and should serve as a guide to any individual occupational therapist, or service, considering how to go about using the occupational therapy professional theory in practice. Although each service describes their own implementation of a specific model, the models chosen just happen to be the ones the practitioners felt were appropriate to their settings and it must be emphasised here that we feel that, if any theory is truly an occupational therapy professional model, then it is possible to use that theory in *any* setting, not just the types of settings described in this book. Thus, Chapters 6 discusses the move towards using the Model of Human Occupation (Kielhofner 1985, 1995, 2002, 2008) in a mental health setting, Chapter 7 discusses the Model of Adaptation through Occupation (Reed and Sanderson 1983, 1992, 1999) in a physical setting and Chapters 8 and 9 discuss the implementation of the Canadian Model of Occupational Performance (Townsend et al 2002), now CMOP-E (Townsend and Polatajko 2007) in a mixed, integrated community and hospital physical setting. However, this is not to say that these are the only settings in which each model can be used.

Chapters 10 and 11 offer a different and wider slant on the use of the theory of occupational therapy in countries where it has been viewed as an emerging profession (both happen to be ex soviet bloc countries) – that is, Chapter 10 asks us to consider the situation of Poland, whilst Chapter 11 discusses the use of theory in occupational therapy in Croatia.

## Investigation into the ways in which occupational therapists and their students learn how to use occupational therapy theory in practice

All of the chapters that narrate the ways in which the professionals have used their theory contain some element of description of the ways in which individual therapists (and by default perhaps students) have learnt how to understand the theory of occupational therapy. However, it is Chapter 2 that reminds us to use our theories and models with caution, that is not as rote learning or lists of instructions for action, but rather as *models for* the profession that offer us guidelines for action, which we must see as needing to be tempered by our own professional judgement. Chapter 4 extends this concept and reminds us to use models of reflection when critiquing our professional practice wisely and to use reflection itself as a way of enhancing our learning about our theory.

## Relationship of the use of theory to the nature of the individual therapist as a person

There are a number of chapters in this book that discuss the factors that influence the individual therapist's use of self in relation to practice and consequently in relation to theory use. However, Chapters 5 and 12 seek to do this most overtly. Finally, Chapter 15 seeks to ask us as individuals to consider our answers to some of the most frequently asked questions related to the use of models. It asks us to determine for ourselves our own view of the place of occupational therapy theory within our own practice.

## Consideration of the place of reflection as a concept to help the occupational therapist get to grips with their understanding of their own theory base

In this book, we are delighted to include a chapter by Della Fish, wherein she takes the opportunity to revisit her 1989 model of reflection – Strands of Reflection (Fish et al 1989) and offers us a new take on the nature of professional thinking and our ways of consequentially reflecting on our theory and ourselves in relation to that theory.

# Conclusion

In this conclusion, we would like to draw the reader's attention to the fact that each chapter begins with a text box of key points that should draw the reader's attention to the chapter's aims and ends (where appropriate) with a list of recommended further reading.

Finally, we would like to acknowledge that the ideas for this book have come from a number of sources. These include our own experiences in practice, our experiences in teaching and using the theory of occupational therapy and, most recently, our experiences of working closely with practitioners in the implementation of models as theory bases for professional action in service settings. The confidence we observed, which many of the practitioners, with whom we worked, gained from using occupational therapy professional models in practice, led us to want to share our thoughts with others; hence, this book was created.

We recognise, of course, that not all members of the profession will necessarily agree with our interpretation of the use of occupational therapy theory in practice, but we hope that this book will be viewed, in the way it is meant, as a serious contribution to the debate.

# References

Fish, D., Twinn, S. and Purr, B. (1989) *How to Enable Learning through Professional Practice: A Cross Profession Investigation of Pre-service Practice*. London: West London Institute.

Kielhofner, G. (1985) *A Model of Human Occupation*. Baltimore: Lippincott, Williams and Wilkins.

Kielhofner, G. (1995) *A Model of Human Occupation*, 2nd edn. Baltimore: Lippincott, Williams and Wilkins.

Kielhofner, G. (2002) *A Model of Human Occupation*, 3rd edn. Baltimore: Lippincott, Williams and Wilkins.

Kielhofner, G. (2008) *A Model of Human Occupation*, 4th edn. Baltimore: Lippincott, Williams and Wilkins.

Reed, K.L. and Sanderson, S.N. (1983) *Concepts of Occupational Therapy*, 2nd edn. Baltimore: Lippincott, Williams and Wilkins.

Reed, K.L. and Sanderson, S.N. (1992) *Concepts of Occupational Therapy*, 3rd edn. Baltimore: Lippincott, Williams and Wilkins.

Reed K.L. and Sanderson, S.N. (1999) *Concepts of Occupational Therapy*, 4th edn. Baltimore: Lippincott, Williams and Wilkins.

Townsend, E., Stanton, S., Law, M., Polatajko, H.J., Baptiste, S., Thompson-Franson, T., Kramer, C., Swedlove, F., Brintnell, S. and Campanile, L. (2002) *Enabling Occupation: An Occupational Therapy Perspective*. Ottawa, ON: CAOT ACE.

Townsend, E.A. and Polatajko, H.J. (2007) *Enabling Occupation II: Advancing an Occupational Therapy Vision for Health, Well-being & Justice through Occupation*. Ottawa, ON: CAOT ACE.

# Section 1

## Theory

# Chapter 2

# Reconfiguring professional thinking and conduct: a challenge for occupational therapists in practice

*Della Fish and Gail Boniface*

---

**Key points**

- Professionalism and defining professional action
- Re-conceptualising professional practice
- The uses and dangers of models for professional practice
- The nature of theory in practice

---

## Introduction

This chapter seeks to encourage occupational therapists to consider their attitude to and use of the theory of their profession. It offers readers a critical lens through which to see and begin to re-vision their professional identity both as individual occupational therapists and as practitioners responsible for shaping their profession's future. In doing so, this chapter underlines the invitation offered in the rest of this book for occupational therapists to rethink and re-conceptualise the theoretical bases on which their professional status currently rests. Such a re-conceptualisation, we hope, will enable occupational therapists to reacquire the confidence to use theory in a manner that will enable them to state clearly their unique and important contribution to the wider territory of health and social care practice, alongside co-professionals such as doctors, nurses, physiotherapists and social workers.

To this end, this chapter considers critically some issues about professions and professionalism in general, whilst at the same time attempts to relate these more general issues to the profession of occupational therapy.

We begin by reviewing what legitimates professionals to be practitioners in the first place and enable occupational therapists to answer 'Yes', when asked if they are members of a profession. We do this, as our experience of occupational therapists is that they regard themselves as members of a *profession* but are not always able to articulate what they mean by that. We continue by critiquing the notion that as

---

*Using Occupational Therapy Theory in Practice*, First Edition. Edited by Gail Boniface and Alison Seymour.
© 2012 Blackwell Publishing Ltd. Published 2012 by Blackwell Publishing Ltd.

professionals our status should depend exclusively on our theoretical knowledge and practical skills. We do view professionalism as containing these two aspects, but suggest that true professionalism is more than that. It requires professionals to harness and use theoretical knowledge and practical skills within their own professional reasoning and intrinsic morality, when working in practice with their clients. (This concept is also explored in Chapter 5.) We then go on to explore the nature of professionalism and the crucial difference between *behaving professionally* and *being a member of a profession*, and what this means about how professionals conduct themselves. This leads to some ideas about theory and the role of practice models in professional practice. As we go along, we offer some definitions of the meanings we accord to certain key terms, which will be taken further in Chapter 3. Throughout, we will present what we view as the practical implications of our ideas for occupational therapy practitioners.

## Professions and professionalism

### What legitimates a practitioner to be a professional?

We all know that entry to professional life (in occupational therapy or any other profession) depends upon the successful completion of an education that has focused on the theory and practice related to preparation for safe practice in our chosen profession. In the Western world, this qualification is usually validated by a university and accredited by an appropriate professional body and the state. But this simple view of the nature of a profession as resting only on the knowledge gained via such an education hides the assumption that we all agree about what would provide the best education and what is the best way to develop further in a professional career. The public has been led to assume that the basis for entry to any profession is an appropriate amount of specialised knowledge that a lay person would not readily know. Thus both factual or *propositional* knowledge (otherwise known as theory or *knowing that*), together with skills or *procedural knowledge* (otherwise known as practice or *knowing how to*), are traditionally regarded as the exclusive essentials to be acquired by the aspiring professional and developed by the qualified practitioner. All this is collectively known as the *epistemological* aspects of professionalism, epistemology being about the nature of knowledge. One of the major issues that occupational therapy has encountered with this trait view (Brint 1993; Hugman 1991) of a profession (the view of the essential nature of factual and specialised knowledge as a definer of a profession) is that occupational therapy in the past had not really owned its own theory, but rather tended to borrow it from areas such as medicine, kinesiology, psychology and sociology. More recently, with the development of a theory course such as occupational science and the practice-based emphasis on occupational analysis as a core skill of occupational therapy, the use of theory in occupational therapy has undergone subtle changes and the theory has begun to be owned by the profession itself. The introduction of models of occupational therapy (discussed further in Chapter 3) as both a theory-based and a practice-based tool has turned the theory of occupational therapy into a much more occupation-centred discipline. Such clearer theoretical definitions have assisted the individual professional to articulate their way of thinking and differentiate occupational therapy from say physiotherapy or social work. However, theory used as dogma can restrict professional practice and shackle the individual professional if not used in what we will refer to as a wise way. Therefore, we argue that rigid use of theory, by applying it unthinkingly to practice, is to distort professionalism. We see specialised knowledge (of theory and of practical skills) as a vital necessity but not, on its own, a sufficient basis for characterising professionalism.

Clearly, what we know (our factual knowledge and our knowledge of skills and procedures) is very important. Thus, for learners seeking to enter a profession, assessments are apparently what count and theory and practice are what is examined. It then follows from this that practitioners' continuing professional development is focused almost solely on updating this knowledge. Interestingly, the same approach is taken by *new professions* seeking public recognition as professions and by so-called semi-professions (Witz 1992) seeking their place in the list of professions. All of these typically seek to deepen and extend their *knowledge* base as *the* magic key to claiming their status as a profession. The curriculum refers to these as knowledge and skills or competencies, and conveniently, these are easily measurable and can be taught through simple instruction and training.

However, this view tends to leave on one side (or even leaves out altogether) the important matter of *who* the professional actually is. By this we mean *what kind of person they are*. This opens up important issues about how professionals actually see (and how they ought to see) themselves and the world around them, how they think, and make judgements, what their values and priorities are, and how cultivated their moral sensibilities are. Along with this go questions about how all the above capacities have been and might be developed or nurtured by education for or within the profession. All this is described as the *ontological* aspects of professionalism where ontology is about the essence or the nature of being. These matters, of course, are not immediately visible and not measurable, though they can be *evidenced* by looking at patterns of development via reflective writing. None of these are either skills or competencies. They are *capacities* that need to be nurtured and developed through education. They certainly cannot be inculcated through training!

It would seem that not only in the United Kingdom particularly but also in much of the Western world, the twentieth century mixture of governmental centralism and the encouragement of the play of market forces have served to emphasise knowledge as the required commodity in professionals and has virtually forced us to neglect the humanity and personhood of the professional. It would seem that the target culture of commercialism and the rule of the market as well as the simplistic conformity demanded by bureaucratic centralism and control have turned knowledge into a commodity. As a commodity, knowledge can be managed by administrators, while the essential humanity of practitioners being difficult to manage is best ignored. (This aspect of professionalism is taken further in Chapter 5 on the use of self.) Yet, ironically, every patient or client, as well as colleagues inside and outside our professions, knows that the professional's ability to establish sound relationships is essential and that therapeutic and collegiate relationships are at the start and the heart of good professional practice in health and social care. In fact, as the users of professionals' services (as the vulnerable clients or patients of a professional), we all know that in practice *epistemology* (theoretical and practical knowledge) and *ontology* (the person you are) both need to be present for sound and successful practice. We regard this to be particularly important in occupational therapy as it consistently claims to be client centred or person centred.

The implications of all this for professions generally and occupational therapy in particular are far reaching. In particular, it raises questions about what the undergraduate curriculum should contain; what counts as professional knowledge (theory and practice); where *theory* comes from, what it is for, and how it can be viewed and used by practitioners; what kind of a person a professional needs to be; how well they can articulate this; and how the profession recognises all this and presents itself to those outside. Professional occupational therapists who can achieve all of this will certainly have no crisis of professional identity and be able to clearly state their professional as well as case-based reasoning.

However, before we consider that in detail, there are other matters that also need to be factored into our thinking, and terms that need to be clarified. Not the least of these is what we might mean by word the *professional* itself.

### What lies beneath the word professional?

Professionalism is an aspect of practice that is significant in shaping good relationships within all health and social care practices. It is recognised by the sick as central to the quality of their care, and is a crucial element in patients' and clients' attitudes to those who care for them. Indeed, a recent Royal College of Physicians' (RCP 2005) report on the importance of medical professionalism saw it as underpinning the trust that the public has in doctors. It stated 'Patients certainly understand the meaning of poor professionalism and associate it with poor medical care'. It continues 'The public is well aware that an absence of professionalism is harmful to their interests' (RCP 2005, p. xi). Professionalism is also a critical factor in the consideration of clinical governance and in medico-legal situations (see Fish and de Cossart 2007).

What then is meant by professionalism? While all those who use the term assume that they know what is involved in being a professional in today's National Health Service (NHS) and social care systems, our professional ideals, aspirations and values that drive practice are far from easy to unearth and express clearly and are often left as implicit or even tacit. For those wishing to explore this more deeply, Chapter 5 of Fish and de Cossart (2007) is a useful starting point. However, the main problem is that today *all* those who work in almost every occupation use the terms *behaving professionally* or *being professional* as a general accolade rather than as a precise descriptor. Thus we learn that a thoroughly planned homicide results in a *very professional murder*, and a well-executed misdemeanour in football is greeted as a *professional foul*! It is also a term used to describe any efficient worker. This is not, of course, to mock those trades-people and merchants who are polite, well dressed, honest, punctual and who, therefore, claim to be professional in their behaviour at work. Rather it is to alert us to the fact that the general word *professional* has changed so much that it no longer carries the particular import it once did.

To recognise the significant distinction between simply *behaving professionally* and being a *member of a profession* is, then, a way of recognising and preserving the more serious and deeper claims that used to be associated with the word. This is not making an elitist suggestion that members of a profession are better than those in other sorts of occupation, because all workers' services are of equal value at the point of need. Rather, what separates members of a profession from all others who earn a living is that their work is different in kind as well as in degree from that of other occupations. Being a *member of a profession* carries with it heavier *moral and social expectations*. Further, many occupations require technical reasoning, but professional practice requires practical reasoning and engagement with a moral mode of practice (see Carr 2004; Fish 2010). Thus if the claim to *be a professional*, made by many health and social care occupations is to be upheld, we need to be clear what this involves.

## What does membership of a profession mean and what are its implications?

Of course there will be many views about what membership of a profession might mean, but what we seek to do in this section is gain a grasp of the general principles involved in the same. As Fish and de Cossart (2007, p. 91) point out 'membership of a profession commits an individual to subscribe to those general values that are found across all professions'.

Members of a profession work in practical human settings and offer a valuable *good*, or well-being, to individuals and society in an altruistic way. Thus, their motivation is at least partly intrinsic and they value the work they do, so that money is not seen as its sole purpose. Professionals seeking to enter a profession must be educated and assessed by members of that profession, because their work is complex, and *in the public interest*. They must also be prepared to engage in life-long development once they begin to practise (see Freidson (1994, 2001) for a further discussion of all of this).

Professional practitioners identify closely with their work and develop intellectual interests in it. Their work involves practical reasoning and takes place in practical settings. This requires the use of esoteric, theoretical knowledge; a research-based high-level skill (none of which a lay person can entirely obtain, totally comprehend or fully evaluate). But there is more to it. It usually involves working with people, who are in some way vulnerable, and thus demands the professional practitioner's acknowledgement of moral and ethical considerations, and involves them in sensitive individual interactions with their patients or clients. This also means that their working context involves the unexpected and the unpredictable and demands the use of their professional judgement, often *on the spot* and always in complex situations. As Fish and de Cossart (2007, p. 91) say: 'The work of a professional is discretionary in nature. This in turn requires that practitioners have self-knowledge and are aware of their own personal and professional values and the values of their profession.' They also point out that:

> 'Confidentiality', 'etiquette' and 'collegiality' are important concepts in the work of a professional practitioner. Their work requires practitioners to operate within the bounds and traditions of the profession through which they are licensed to practice. Such traditions have been developed over a long period in response to the demands and values of society. Professional bodies are the guardians of these standards, and as such are regulatory.
>
> (Fish and de Cossart 2007, p. 91)

Thus, whilst it is true that we live in a changing world and that in the early twenty-first century, the performance target culture has eroded some of professionals' traditional ways of working and being this does not release them from the moral duty to keep under review their roles, responsibilities and obligations to their patients or clients. Indeed, as many professions have already recognised, they will fail the public if they allow these crucial characteristics to be obscured and undervalued. That is why the curriculum for those seeking entry to any profession has to raise awareness of these matters, and all members of a profession need to have clarified for themselves where they stand, and have a clear idea of their implications for themselves and for their profession.

This is particularly important, but difficult, given that the predominant public discourse of health and social care practitioners and their teachers are shaped by a technical rational view of practice. In Fish (2010, p. 192), this was described as foregrounding 'standards', 'competencies' and 'quality assurance activities', which are designed to control and shape professional behaviour from outside practice. However, the profession, itself, often goes beyond such technical rational views of professional action and will include profession-specific thinking and morality. In occupational therapy, this can be seen in the subtle differences between the educational standards the Health Professions Council (HPC 2009) requires of occupational therapy curricula and the expectations of the College of Occupational Therapists (COT 2008) of the same curricula. Due to the regulatory nature of the organisations emphasising technical rationality, this means that:

> when professionals discuss their work publicly, they emphasise technical expertise where evidence-based practice achieves the highest accolade, and proof of the quality of care lies in fitting individual cases into patterns created by the analysis of trends and measurements.
>
> (Fish 2010, p. 192)

Fish (2010) also pointed out that technical rationalism *claims* to be *the way* to ensure patient safety. This emphasises the need to learn and apply general skills and rules to an individual case. Such a way of working offers the practitioner the excuse to refrain from engaging in morally committed action, but brings into question the technical rational way of working's compatibility with patient, client or person-centred care.

Technical rationalism, as Dunne (2005, p. 373) pointed out, is 'closely related to modern science' but 'has roots in Western philosophy, traceable back to the Socratic valorisation of techne'. *Techne* is Aristotle's term for the disposition to act in a rule-governed way that is guided by 'the general aim of making or producing some object or artifact' (Carr 2009, p. 60). This view:

> puts a premium on 'objectivity' and detachment, suppressing the context-dependence of first-person experience in favour of a third-person perspective which yields generalised findings in accordance with clearly formulated, publicly agreed procedures. These procedures give an indispensible role to operations of observation and measurement, . . . and the adoption of a language maximally freed from the possibilities of misinterpretation by its being maximally purged of the need for interpretation itself.
>
> (Dunne 2005, p. 373)

The all-pervasive control of this mindset over thinking in the Western world has restricted this view into 'the only way of seeing'. Yet other forms of seeing and thinking do exist, and always have, as Aristotle pointed out. These are associated with other ways of 'seeing ourselves and the world around us' that lead to different ways of acting (see Carr 2009, p. 60). This means, as Fish (2010, pp. 192–193) points out:

> where techne disposes us to be governed by rules and is about instrumental action (needing the support of trainers), *episteme* disposes us to seek truth and involves contemplative action (needing philosophical and logical dialogue with teachers), and *phronesis* is the disposition to do what is best in individual cases, which leads to morally committed action (and needs the nurturing of educational *praxis*).

And in their practice, *phronesis* is actually what most professionals seek to embrace. They make decisions about what is best for a particular person at a given time. They do not just follow protocols or models blindly. As Fish (2010, p. 193) continues, professionals:

> engage in interpreting the individual patient's humane needs and adjusting the general scientific clinical solution of what is right for a given disease [or patient's rehabilitation] to what seems to be the best for this particular person. This often involves creating new knowledge in practice rather than applying known solutions to practice. Thus, in their work, professionals engage not in technical rationality but in practical reasoning (phronesis) and morally committed action (praxis).

Thus, ironically, while professionals often talk as if they practise rationally, and seek to defend their practice in clear-cut and absolute terms, they actually use interpretation and professional judgement (acting with discretion on the patient or client's behalf) and thus engage in practical professional rationality, not technical rationality.

Many occupational therapists within both health and social care, work alongside or in positions of management over unqualified support staff such as carers, technical instructors or assistants. If professional action could simply be pared down to technical rational action, then these support workers who are *unqualified* (in contrast to the full professional) could simply work instead of the professional at carrying out clearly defined technical actions. However, that does not happen and in reality such support workers actually work under the guidance or direction of the professional occupational therapist. How could this be justified if the professional occupational therapist were not perceived to be offering a different type of intervention to the technical rational one of the support worker? However, this question is not as clear cut as it may appear and the differences between such unqualified (in professional terms) support staff is often blurred and attractive to the employing organisation, as a support worker is obviously not as expensive to employ as a qualified practitioner. This is why professionals need to formulate their personal philosophy and develop the courage to act according to their professional conscience (informed by an understanding of principled autonomy, see Winch 2006). Some resources for exploring this further are available in Fish and de Cossart (2007), and some means of reflecting on this are to be found in Chapter 4.

Therefore, being a member of a profession is not about *behaving professionally*, because many people in many occupations can claim to do that by demonstrating that they act with general propriety. By contrast, membership of a profession is about conducting oneself on the basis of practical professional rationality, within the traditions of one's profession. This calls upon moral sensibilities and the capacity to make wise judgements, on behalf of the vulnerable, in complex situations.

## How professionals use models in practice: thinking like a professional

It will be clear from what we have said so far, that *thinking like a professional* is not about automatically applying theory, protocols or models to practice, but rather about using them with discretion and only where appropriate, within practice. As we have already indicated, this involves interpretation of the individual client's or patient's needs. But it also presupposes an understanding of the nature of theory and of theoretical protocols and models. This brings with it the need to understand:

- the nature of theory, the range of kinds of theory, and its relationship to practice;
- the relationship between models and the reality they purport to explain; and
- the role of models within theory and practice.

It also demands, within all this, a firm grasp of the dangers of models.

## The nature of theory

Theory is not simple fact, and the term *theory* does not have one simple meaning. It may mean a set of statements or principles devised to explain a group of facts or phenomena, especially one that has been repeatedly tested or is widely accepted. In this sense, it offers explanatory statements, accepted principles, and methods of analysis, as opposed to practice, and involves abstract reasoning (and often, speculation). However, the word *theory* can sometimes mean a belief or principle that guides action or assists comprehension or judgment. Quite often it is an assumption based on limited information or knowledge or a conjecture. Usually it is an organised system of accepted knowledge that applies in a variety of circumstances to explain a specific set of phenomena involving *hypotheses* and *systematic modelling*.

There being various kinds of theory, it is important to distinguish between them and act within practice accordingly. Thus, *formal theory* is a set of ideas in a logical system (themselves a mixture of beliefs, values and assumptions) formulated and argued for publicly, commonly known and acknowledged. However, it is also important to remember that formal theory is not a *proven fact* even when it rests on research reported as absolute fact!

By contrast, *personal theories* are privately held ideas that do not necessarily hang coherently together, but consist of a mixture of beliefs, values and assumptions, which are untested in the public arena, and heavily influence our practices and determine how we interpret the world and shape our encounters with people, situations and ideas. Those theories that we *say* (and believe) influence us or our thinking and actions are known as *espoused theories*, those that actively govern our actions and decisions are our *theories in use*. These two can sometimes be mismatched and this causes us to ask: do we always do what we say (or believe) we should do? In occupational therapy our espoused theories are based on the client/patient's occupations, but how often are our actions a true reflection of this? The relationship of theory to practice is also more complex than at first appears. Theory can be *applied to practice*; can enlighten practice; can be developed within practice (as you go); and can be developed by those who look at practice and *theorise it*. When theory is *applied to practice*, it is likely that technical reasoning is involved and that the *theory* has been constructed by someone other than a practitioner, and handed down to those *on the ground*. This may mean that it less than perfectly matches with what is found in the practitioner's context and particular needs. Theory can enlighten practice when it is used to prompt practitioners to think for themselves about their practice and see more in it through the reflection guided by the theory. Theory can be developed within practice by practitioners who think openly and critically about their actions and recognise for themselves new meanings within their practice. Practice can be *theorised* by those who start by observing a range of practices and developing new ways of generalising about it. Models (which are a form of theory) may have begun from the observation of practice, but these observations are then interpreted into general principles and offered in a structure that make them readily applicable by practitioners. There are problems with this, however as the next section will discuss.

## The nature of models and their hidden dangers

Theoretical ideas offered by models are often woolly and unstable, and further, definitions of a number of terms in occupational therapy are not just woolly and unstable but contradictory (Duncan 2006; Creek 2003). This woolliness is addressed in Chapter 3 of this book that offers definitions of terms often used interchangeably within occupational therapy. One thing that is certain is that models are crude representations of complex reality and as such *can* help practitioners to interpret reality when used within client and patient practice. However, occupational therapy models offer theoretical constructs of the way someone has seen a part of their world – in this instance, their interpretation of the theory and practice of occupational therapy. In that sense they are neither as objective nor as absolute as they can appear to be. They provide *as if* pictures of a defined part of life – someone's picture that asks us to see reality as if it were like this (often stripped of what are labelled as irrelevant details). Therefore, it is very important not to mistake the picture for the real thing.

Often, models will claim to provide scientific, law-like, generalisations of the world and when they do so, this usually means that they are reductionist and interpretative. They reduce the complexities of real life so that we can (apparently) see the main bones of it (as interpreted by the theorist) and deduce the principles and laws running behind it. In this way, theorists identify trends and patterns and then harden them into scientific and apparently objective theory. It is a short but dangerous step from this to assume that as practitioners we should take on and *apply* this theory to our practice. Such theory is, after all, only an interpretation and our practice, as we see it, may be more complex than the theory allows for. Models then are one person's or a team's particular choice of what to remove from the complexity of reality they have studied, what to count as *the bare bones* of it, and, therefore, what to leave out of it. They are attempts at constructing a view of 'reality' (but it is one view) and they work on valid patterns and memorable (or sometimes slick) ways of exhibiting data. Having presented the negative side of models, and our consequential suggestion that we should treat them with caution, we will now offer a more positive view of models. We consider that there are different types of models available to professional occupational therapists and that they are not all unhelpful to practitioners.

## The role of models within theory and practice

As discussed in the preceding text, models can offer a variety of kinds of *as if* pictures. These can be operational, structural or conceptual pictures. The operational ones (*models of how to practice*) tend to offer us a potentially rigid way of doing something, whereas the structural and conceptual ones (*models for practice*) can enlighten how we see practice. It is important to distinguish between these models *of* and models *for* practice within occupational therapy.

Models *of* (e.g. models of health care) are the invention by theorists of general laws and principles (which are actually hypotheses) aimed at explaining a holistic phenomenon to be applied to practice by practitioners. The ideas may have emerged initially as a result of an examination of some aspects of practice, but they have been built upon theoretically by theorists until they have reached a holistic entity that encapsulates all elements of the thing modelled, and to a level at which generalisations can be made and the future can be predicted and prophesied. But all this is often further and further from practitioners' experience of current practice. Such models treat human practices scientifically, which is illogical, and assume a level of objectivity that cannot exist within the complexity of human enterprises and particularly in individualised and person-centred occupational therapy practice. Indeed, the assertions and assumptions that imposed *models of*, encapsulate, are often readily seen to be at variance with *reality*, experienced or observed in situ. An example would be *a comprehensive model of human behaviour*, when of course there can never be such a thing (see, e.g., Steinitz and Goldman 1997).

By contrast, *models for* are often models for practitioners to use to explore and illuminate their practice, or perhaps guide it loosely. They demand less adherence to one particular view of practice and as such can be useful to wise practitioners who have matured into enquirers into their own practice. This is because wise practitioners recognise the particularity of practice, which requires them in the end to use their own thought and judgement.

## Conclusion

The 'price of the employment of models is eternal vigilance' (see Braithwaite quoted in Kerr 1968, p. 86). Models can make those in practice look for specific examples of the general laws they offer, but in doing so, they often cause practitioners to mistake the relationship between the general and the particular. For example, occupational therapists using a theoretical model without thinking could blindly insist on dealing with every individual with a certain disability in the same way because the theory suggests a particular course of action.

In order to avoid this, firstly we have to ask: are we willing to accept the operational definitions of the models as representative of the reality we encounter in practice? Then we have to ask whether our particular practice will sensibly yield to this model as a whole (treating it as a *model of*), or whether instead it is a model that might help us to enlighten our own view of our own practice situation (treating it as a *model for*). We also have to ask whether we would be better attempting to theorise our own practice – to understand it by seeing what is in the practice and recognising patterns within it. It is worth remembering that, unlike given *models of*, our own theorising is always open to re-vision and re-interpretation. However, as most of the occupational therapy models discussed within the professional literature are holistic and occupational in nature (as is occupational therapy), we feel they offer a more general view of professional practice and viewing them as *models for* occupational therapy, which can enable individual occupational therapists to investigate and reflect on their own individualised practice, is a more professionally helpful way forward.

## References

Brint, S. (1993) Eliot Friedson's contribution to the sociology of professions. *Work and Occupations*, 20(3), 259–278.

Carr, D. (2004) Rival Conceptions of Practice in Education and Teaching. In: *Education and Practice: Upholding the Integrity of Teaching and Learning*, eds J. Dunne and P. Hogan. Oxford: Blackwell Publishing Ltd.

Carr, W. (2009). Practice without theory? A postmodern perspective on educational practice. In: *Understanding and Researching Professional Practice*, ed. B. Green, pp. 55–64. Rotterdam: Sense Publications.

College of Occupational Therapists (COT) (2008) *College of Occupational Therapists Pre-registration Education Standards*. London: College of Occupational Therapists.

Creek, J. (2003) *Occupational Therapy Defined as a Complex Intervention*. London: College of Occupational Therapists.

Duncan, A.S. (ed.) (2006) *Foundations for Practice in Occupational Therapy*, 4th edn. Edinburgh: Elsevier Churchill Livingstone.

Dunne, J. (2005) An intricate fabric: understanding the rationality of practice. *Pedagogy, Culture and Society* 13(3), 367–389.

Fish, D. (2010) Learning to practise interpretively: exploring and developing practical rationality. In: *Education for Future Practice*, eds J. Higgs, D. Fish, I. Goulter, S. Loftus, J. Reid and F. Trede. Rotterdam: Sense Publications.

Fish, D. and de Cossart, L. (2007) *Developing the Wise Doctor*. London: Royal Society of Medicine Press.

Freidson, E. (1994) *Professionalism Reborn: Theory, Prophecy and Policy*. Oxford: Polity Press.

Freidson, E. (2001) *Professionalism: the Third Way*. Oxford: Polity Press.

Health Professions Council. (2009) *Standards of Education and Training*. United Kingdom: Health Professions Council.

Hugman, R. (1991) *Power in Caring Professions*. Basingstoke: Macmillan Education.

Kerr, J.F. (ed.) (1968) *Changing the Curriculum*. London: University of London Books Ltd. (Unibooks).

Royal College of Physicians (RCP) (2005) *Doctors in Society, Medical Professionalism in a Changing World: Report of a Working Party*. London: Royal College of Physicians.

Steinitz, R. and Goldman, S. (1997) Towards a comprehensive theoretical model of human behavior. *Journal of Social and Evolutionary Systems* 20(2), 185–189. Available online 21 April 2002.

Winch, C. (2006) *Education, Autonomy and Critical Thinking*. London: Routledge.

Witz, A. (1992) *Professions and Patriarchy*. New York: Routledge.

## Further reading

Carr, D. (2004) Rival conceptions of practice in education and teaching, In: *Education and Practice: Upholding the Integrity of Teaching and Learning*, eds J. Dunne and P. Hogan. Oxford: Blackwell Publishing Ltd.

Fish, D. (2010) Learning to practise interpretively: exploring and developing practical rationality, In: *Education for future practice*, eds J. Higgs, D. Fish, I. Goulter, S. Loftus, J. Reid and F. Trede. Rotterdam: Sense Publications.

Fish, D. and de Cossart, L. (2007) *Developing the Wise Doctor*. London: Royal Society of Medicine Press.

Freidson, E. (1994) *Professionalism Reborn: Theory, Prophecy and Policy*. Oxford: Polity Press.

## Chapter 3

# Defining occupational therapy theory
*Gail Boniface*

---

**Key points**

- Occupational therapy can be defined as a profession for many reasons, including its unique theory base
- Theory terms are numerous and can be confusing
- The relationship of theory concepts to one another is more important than the names of those concepts
- Theory forms an umbrella for occupational therapists to shelter under where the model of the profession forms the sturdy umbrella spines

---

## Introduction

This chapter discusses the nature of professionalism, as it relates to occupational therapy, along with the way in which the profession's theory assists in defining that professionalism. It also discusses the terms usually used to describe the components of that professionalism (see also Chapter 2). Thus, it offers my definitions of those terms and their relationship to one another, which I have found to be useful in practice. It concludes by offering an overview of some of the main theories upon which occupational therapy bases itself and a brief description of the models I regard as central to our profession.

## What might make occupational therapy a profession?

According to most occupational therapists, and the state in many countries, occupational therapy is a profession. Its members are often registered by the state, and as a consequence, the profession (or rather an individual practitioner within it) is required to engage in activities, which will demonstrate suitability to maintain a place on the state register. These activities include reflection, engaging in continuing professional development, following codes of conduct and utilising theory appropriately. In Britain,

---

*Using Occupational Therapy Theory in Practice*, First Edition. Edited by Gail Boniface and Alison Seymour.
© 2012 Blackwell Publishing Ltd. Published 2012 by Blackwell Publishing Ltd.

such state registration also requires adherence to the expected competencies of practitioners (Health Professions Council 2007) and consequently, the detailing to the profession, of the standards for its educational courses (Health Professions Council 2009). For an occupational therapist, the content of the profession's required activities or skills form part of the profession's identity and are aspects that differentiate it and its practitioners both from other professionals and from support staff in the workplace. This can narrow the focus of the profession into seeing skills as the centre of professional practice. That is, this view tends to concentrate on the competencies of the practitioner, sometimes to the detriment of their professional identity. These competencies can then force the therapist to focus on the skills to be learnt or improved by the client, rather than their occupational behaviour that results from those skills. Such skills concentration is often derived from an analysis of *individual* occupational therapists' *behaviour* (which must be *seen* to occur and is, therefore, easily measured). Relying simply on the behaviour of individual therapists to define professional identity can distort the way in which occupational therapy is viewed as a profession. What such a competency-based approach to professional practice omits or overlooks is all the invisible elements of what is involved in being an occupational therapist, and all the aspects of it that do not easily yield to measurement. In particular, what can occur (in all professions) is that the emphasis on competencies can cause us to overlook the core essence of professional practice such as individual professional judgement, the moral nature of professional practice (as discussed in Chapter 2) and the use of profession-specific theory.

Taking the above into account, it is important to consider *why* occupational therapy is a profession, rather than simply asserting it. In order to do so, it is important to consider a number of issues; beginning with consideration of the sociological view of what makes a job a profession and by so doing I will offer usable definitions of professional theory terminology.

## Theory development and the profession of occupational therapy

The desire for the status of profession and the aspirations of *job holders* to attain the title of *professionals* is well documented in sociology literature (Hugman 1991; Witz 1992; Brint 1993). Professions are also classified as such, via a number of different descriptions, which often include the demonstrable traits of the profession and relate to issues such as power, professional closure and patriarchy (Witz 1992; Brint 1993). Although somewhat embedded in the 1950s and 1960s (Brint 1993), the trait view of professions still has some resonance within the profession of occupational therapy. Often the traits of a profession can be seen as follows:

- Professional autonomy
- Registration and standard setting
- Altruism
- A discrete body of knowledge owned by the profession

Whilst all of the above could be claimed to be inherent in occupational therapy, it is the profession's discrete body of knowledge that has always caused the most debate. As a profession, occupational therapy for a long time tended to borrow or use the knowledge that is more commonly associated with other professions, such as social work or medicine; and tended to lack its own. To add to this theory issue, where it has made attempts to define its knowledge base, it has often had difficulties agreeing on the definitions of the terms with which that knowledge is associated. The next section will offer my views on those terms.

### Theory terms: a lack of clarity?

According to Smith (1992): 'Theorising is simply the name given to the process of reflecting on practice' (p. 388). This book is concerned with the process of developing the professional occupational therapist through their understanding and use of theory and consequently their own understanding of their professional thinking. The professional thinking referred to in the previous sentence is obviously clinical reasoning, but is also at the deeper level of reflecting on professional action and its relationship to the practitioner's professional identity. Many of the theories of occupational therapy are concerned with defining and categorising the issue of occupation and occupational engagement. Many other theories that occupational therapists use are at a basic skill level and can make it hard to see the occupational aspects of the occupational therapist's everyday actions.

The interesting thing about occupational therapy is that its tradition (or foundational knowledge) is known to all practitioners, but not necessarily *overtly used or articulated* by all practitioners. The foundational knowledge of occupational therapy is undoubtedly rooted in the understanding, analysis and use of occupation to enable clients to deal with or compensate for underlying conditions and disabilities. There are, of course, pressing reasons offered for not basing our practice in occupation and rather in those conditions or disabilities. However, these can often be imposed from outside the profession by the organisations within which we work and do not really sit comfortably with the profession's tradition.

However the theory is viewed, it cannot be denied that there are a confusing number of words used to describe the theory of occupational therapy and an equally confusing number of definitions of those words. There are words such as philosophy, paradigm, organismic and mechanismic paradigm, model, meta-model, approach, theory and frame of reference. Last, but not the least is the actual purpose of professional existence – the practice of the profession. In occupational and professional literature (Mosey 1981; Reed 1984; Hagedorn 2001; Tyrer and Steinberg 2005; Duncan 2006; Turpin and Iwama 2011), there are a large number of ways of interpreting these terms. So is it any wonder that, on occasions, we as individual professionals become confused about how to use the concepts championed by these terms in our practice? This section attempts to define these professional terms in a way that has proved useful in practice for occupational therapists and students with whom I have worked. It is hoped that the definitions offered will help occupational therapists to make sense of the occupational core of the profession, whilst at the same time enabling them to use other related or even non-related theories for the benefit of their clients. It goes without saying that these interpretations may be viewed as contentious. They are offered here in the spirit of adding to rather than settling the debate around definitions. They also constitute a genuine attempt on my part to offer some workable and usable definitions of the terms, which may assist occupational therapists in their practice.

## Definitions of theory terms

In this section, I have chosen to define five aspects or components that I feel are contained to a greater or lesser extent in explaining the theory of occupational therapy. The components are as follows:

- Paradigm
- Philosophy
- Model
- Approach
- Practice

The definitions offered in this section will be used throughout this book. As I have indicated in the preceding text, defining these terms is not as simple a task as it may appear at first. Many of the definitions offered elsewhere (Hagedorn 2001; Creek 2003; Duncan 2006; Kielhofner and Forsyth 2006; Cole and Tuffano 2008) can be viewed as contentious. As Duncan (2006) says: 'it is important to remain mindful that specific terms are still being used by different people in different ways' (p. 61). For example, the occupational therapy reference dictionary offers a confusing picture of synonymous definitions by referring to a paradigm as: 'an organising interaction. A pattern, example or model' (Jacobs and Jacobs 2009, p. 182) and a model as: 'An approach, a framework or structure that organises knowledge' (Jacobs and Jacobs 2009, p. 152). In order to clarify the stance of this book, I offer here my view of both the definitions of the terms and the relationship or interaction between the concepts they represent, which in my experience works in practice. At the end of this definitions section, the concept of this relationship between the terms in practice is offered as an umbrella for locating and sheltering occupational therapy practice.

## Paradigm

According to Reed and Sanderson (1992, p. 38), a *paradigm* is a 'most comprehensive belief and value system' that can be viewed as the underpinning philosophical view of man upon which a profession bases itself. Some contradictory examples are the mechanistic versus humanistic or reductionist versus holistic paradigms. However, according to Hagedorn (1992, p. 6), others view a paradigm as performing the function of providing 'a single statement of the fundamental principles on which a profession is based'. I view this definition as being more in tune with my definition of philosophy. Thus, my definition of paradigm offered here tends to agree with that of Reed and

Sanderson (1992) and views a paradigm more as a *world view* (Weltanschauung) or the basic but grand underlying belief system, which members of a profession generally adhere to. In the case of occupational therapy, that is generally humanistic and holistic. It is also unlikely to shift or become revolutionised (Kuhn 1996) within the profession of occupational therapy as it is perhaps the most fundamentally held belief system of the profession: That occupational therapy believes in the need to view people in a holistic and person-centred way; a view it shares with a number of professions such as social work.

Viewing a paradigm as such a large-scale belief system for a profession means that it can then be shared with other like-minded professions. It can then be used to reason around the disagreements that can occur with other professions that base themselves within a different paradigm; for example the very different views encompassed by the medical and the social view of disability. Thus, although the paradigm begins to point towards the nature of a profession and an explanation of its way of working, it does not clearly define a profession, but rather attempts to encapsulate its general attitude. As this general attitude is also shared with others and does not belong exclusively to occupational therapy, what is needed, if an individual profession is to be defined, is another layer of theory: A layer that offers a more individualised (to the profession) view of the nature of the profession. I view this more individualised concept as the *philosophy* of the profession.

### Philosophy

The philosophy of a profession can be seen as a broad-based theory, which puts forward the profession's (rather than as in the paradigm, a group of professions') general beliefs. The philosophy is not generally well defined, but is an indicator of a profession's way of thinking, rather than an expression of its larger belief system (paradigm), which it shares with others. In contrast to the paradigm, then, the philosophy does indeed belong to and begin to define the profession. In occupational therapy, the philosophy discusses the concept of occupation, person centredness and the environment within which people carry out occupations. It also suggests a feeling that engagement in occupations can improve or overcome illness and disability. Occupational therapy's philosophy basically follows a problem-solving route (assessment, planning, intervention, evaluation – often, erroneously in my opinion, referred to as the occupational therapy process) and has as its central tenet the fact that: 'man *(meaning mankind)* through the use of his hands as they are energised by mind and will can influence the state of his own health' (Reilly 1962, p. 88). Occupational therapists then act in a problem-solving way WITH the client's *active* participation via occupations or activities or to overcome difficulties with carrying out occupations within their environment.

As we can see, this philosophy is very occupationally based and helpful in determining the main business of the occupational therapist. What it does not do, however, is offer anything more specific for us to use. It is a woolly statement (although nowhere near as woolly as a paradigm) rather than any kind of guide, or tool, for use in practice. It is nevertheless a statement that is essential to keep us all on the occupational rather than any other track. Helpful though our philosophy (in a woolly sense!) may be, what we need in addition to the philosophy of our profession is something a little more concrete, that perhaps points us towards certain actions or at least away from others. Something we can use to begin to organise our professional thinking whilst at the same time offering us a flexibility to use our own professional judgement, artistry and professional reasoning. This next level I view as the model of the profession.

## Model

> All professions have a model that serves as the basis for practice. Such a model may be publicly stated or part of the unarticulated tradition of a profession.
>
> (Mosey 1981, p. 41)

A model can be seen as a theoretical definition of a profession, which is more concrete than its philosophy. A model tends to point towards certain action and is owned by the profession alone (e.g. Mosey 1981; Kielhofner 1985). It is a way of guiding action (the practice) that is much more practical than the philosophy. Even so, it does not preclude the use of approaches (see in the following text), but rather directs the way in which a specific profession may use approaches. It tends to provide that specific profession with its own, unique framework into which approaches can be slotted, if and when they are relevant.

However, not all models are clearly stated: 'ideas often are not well articulated, but rather are shown at the level of "belief"' (Mosey 1981, p. 57). For some years occupational therapy lived with a certain inarticulacy in this respect, but *has* developed its own models. As yet, *no one* model has emerged as the front-runner and indeed that may not even be desirable. As again, according to Mosey (1981), professional models should not stagnate, but should evolve with time in order to respond to societal changes and demands.

A model to summarise, can be viewed and used as a basis for practice, but it offers us more of an outline for our professional action, not a rulebook to be directly applied to practice. It should also be unique to the profession and as such can be used as a framework upon which to base the activities of our profession and against which to measure the success of its intervention (outcomes).

Therefore, in order to bridge the gap between the model(s) and the practice of a profession, a further link needs to be found. This link can be regarded as approaches to intervention.

## Approaches to intervention

An approach can be seen as the interface between the profession's own unique model(s) and its practice. An approach does not only belong to one profession *but to many*. It is the therapist's chosen method of putting his/her model into practice. It will often be used by others, but in different ways, depending on their models. It may be the agreed method of action for all team members (e.g. Behaviourism and Bobath), but will, or should, be practised in different ways by different professions. For example, if a therapist adopts the Cognitive Behavioural Approach when practising occupational therapy with a specific client, he or she is *not* practising cognitive behaviourism, but using that approach within the framework of a model of occupational therapy. An approach is not a definition (as the profession's model is) of the individual profession that might use the approach. To tread that path is a very dangerous way to travel and leads to role erosion rather than the role blurring required in teamwork. Therefore, the approach is a guide rather than a recipe for action and fits into the individual profession's model rather than dictating it. One way of regarding approaches is to view them as a practical link between the model of a profession and its practitioners' action. There are many different approaches to intervention, which influence (and occasionally dominate) occupational therapy. However, rarely is one approach followed slavishly to the exclusion of all others. Even where a specific approach (e.g. some neuro-developmental ones) excludes another, by its very nature, the occupational therapist often adapts and changes the approach to fit in with their model of occupational therapy. The use of a number of approaches at any one time is often termed 'eclecticism' or in a more derogatory manner 'jack of all trades'. However, there would seem to be *absolutely nothing wrong with eclecticism as long as the therapist claiming to be eclectic understands the theory behind the different approaches they are dipping into.* In order to remain an occupational therapist when using any, or indeed a number of approaches to intervention, the therapist simply needs to use them under the umbrella of an occupational therapy model (see Figure 3.1), otherwise the therapist's eclecticism can appear to be a lack of understanding of the approaches' theories or the theory of occupational therapy.

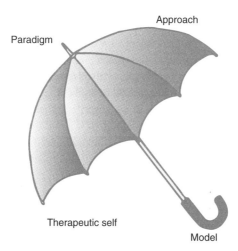

**Figure 3.1**  The Umbrella of Professional Practice. The handle and stem of the umbrella are the sound, sturdy and trusted model of the profession. The spines or ribs of the umbrella are the approaches that are used to put the model into practice and which cannot be held aloft without the model. The fabric of the umbrella (which keeps the rain off the professional) is the therapist themself and their use of self, whilst the point of the umbrella is the paradigm to which the professional generally adheres.

Finally, in this section, it should be noted that all of the theory terms discussed in the preceding text mean nothing without the practice of the profession.

### Practice

Practice is the carrying out of the profession's roles, guided by approaches, defined by a model and influenced by a philosophy, by an individual professional who generally believes a particular overview of the world (paradigm). In reality, the distinct roles of different professions may not be quite so distinct, especially in inter- or multi-disciplinary teamwork. The professional who bases their practice on a sound professional theoretical base will be able to act outside their professional model, but will always be aware of the occasions when they are doing so and are less likely to define their profession through someone else's theory (e.g. an approach to intervention) or view of their action. Once again Figure 3.1 illustrates the inter-relationship of these terms, which I view as being as important as their definitions.

Section 'Models of occupational therapy' offers an overview of the models that belong to the profession of occupational therapy, for further information on each individual model, the reader is directed to the original authors of the model as recommended at the end of this chapter.

## Models of occupational therapy

In occupational therapy over the past 40 years there have been a number of professional models suggested for use in practice. These have been greeted with views, which ranged from scepticism as to their usefulness, suspicion as to the need for them, or evangelical desire to adopt them. However they may be viewed, I believe that models grow (with the undoubted nurturing of academics) from practice and that each model of occupational therapy currently in use or under review has evolved in relationship to, as a consequence of, or alongside another. After all, they are all related to the profession and all stem from the profession's philosophy. Hence, it is not surprising that all models contain similar ideas, expressed in differing ways. It should also be noted that changes in the model(s) can occur as a result of changes in practice at the practice (therapist) level just as at the academic thinking level. Hence the common cry of therapists when investigating a *new* model 'but we've always done that'. I often find myself agreeing with such a statement, but when asked to demonstrate such action, therapists are frequently unable to do so in a clear manner and would perhaps benefit from using a model for the profession to clarify their professional thinking.

A number of professional models of occupational therapy can be seen as having developed in a hierarchical manner as individual occupational therapists struggled to theorise on and articulate the existing and unique ideas of the profession. It is proposed here that A Model of Purposeful Activity (Fidler and Fidler 1963) was the first and a Model of Adaptive Skills and the Biopsychosocial Model (Mosey 1968, 1974, 1980, 1986) the second modern attempts to define models of occupational therapy. While a Model of Human Occupation (Kielhofner 1985), a Model of Adaptation through Occupation (Reed and Sanderson 1983) and the Canadian Model of Occupational Performance (CAOT 1991; Townsend and Polatajko 2007) form more current, later, model descriptions for the profession of occupational therapy. There are of course others, such as the Person Environment Occupation Model (Law et al 1996) – often connected with the Canadian – and the Kawa River Model (Iwama 2006), which in my opinion is more akin to a general philosophy and not a model of the profession of occupational therapy.

The next section briefly outlines the history and development of models of the profession defined as such above. As stated previously, for further information on the models, the reader is recommended to access the original writers' descriptions, as this section simply intends to offer an overview in order to provide a context for this book's practice led chapters on using models in context.

### *A Model of Purposeful Activity* Fidler & Fidler (1963)

This *model* is based on the belief that purposeful activities provide incentives and opportunities for individuals to achieve mastery of themselves, and thereby add to their sense of competence. It views the individual as capable of controlling their destiny (and by implication health) via their occupations and that they can influence the state of their health through the things they do. It closely considers the meaning and use of activities to an individual. Although it *could* be viewed as a model of occupational therapy, I would see Fidler and Fidler's (1963) *model* as:

1. an extension to Reilly's (1962) statement of the philosophy of occupational therapy; or
2. a definition of activity analysis utilised in all other models of occupational therapy.

As a *model* in its own right, it tends to remain a little vague and as such could be viewed at either end of a profession's structure, that is its philosophy or its practical application (as noted in 1 and 2 in the preceding text).

### *Model of Adaptive Skills* (Anne Cronin Mosey 1986)

Mosey's *model* of adaptive skills is based on the belief that humans are continually adapting their actions and behaviours to the environment in which they find themselves. It is based on a developmental framework in which adaptation occurs sequentially and is dependent on the skills and sub-skills acquired earlier. In the *model*, individuals acquire discrete skills in different skills' areas over a developmental period and alter or adapt the way in which they *use* those skills in different circumstances. Thus the real skill is that of adaptation rather than the acquisition of small sub-skills. The adaptive skills are developmental in nature and are split into sequential sub-skills, all of which need to be mastered in order to allow the individual to modify the skill, that is make it an *adaptive* one. Mosey (1986) accepts that it is not always possible for an individual to acquire all the necessary discrete skills. She notes that at times it may be possible to cope with a lack of skill by learning splinter skills, which compensate for the lack, but in so doing, she argues (1986), the emphasis is changed from a developmental to an acquisitional (or compensatory) one. Although discussed as a *model*, Mosey's own argument that the learning of splinter skills is justified if the framework changes from a developmental to a compensatory one, illustrates the likelihood that by this book's definition, the adaptive skills *model* is actually a developmental approach. As such it, therefore, does not offer a model of occupational therapy by this book's definition, but a useful slant on development.

Although the two models discussed in the preceding text influence our way of thinking as occupational therapists, they either do not offer much practical guidance for occupational therapy action (Fidler and Fidler 1963) or are more akin to an approach (Mosey 1986). Thus, they are not commonly used as a model of occupational therapy per se in practice but are rather seen as therapy influences. The following three models, however, are indeed used in practice, as subsequent chapters will demonstrate.

## A Model of Adaptation through Occupation (Reed and Sanderson originally 1983)

Reed and Sanderson place great emphasis on the environment in which the individual carries out occupations, the occupations in terms of their relevance to the individual, the skill levels required to master the occupation and the adaptations the individual must make either to himself or to his environment in order to successfully carry out the occupation. The type of words they use indicate the influence on their thinking of Fidler and Fidler (1963), Mosey (1968, 1986), and perhaps Kielhofner (1985) who was developing the Model of Human Occupation at a similar time. Reed and Sanderson's (1983, 1992, 1999) model is based on their basic assumption that:

> the study and management of the purposeful occupations (activities) in which humans engage is the unique feature of Occupational Therapy that separates the knowledge base from all other professions'.
>
> (Reed and Sanderson 1983, p. 7)

They believe that damage to the individual (illness, disability), a disruptive environment and an imbalance of types of occupation create an inability to cope and cause further deterioration in health. There are strong developmental elements in the model, leading from primitive (original) reflexes through the development of individual skills to successful adaptive performance of occupations. By adaptive, they mean the individual adapts or alters themselves and/or the environment in which they carry out occupations in order to attain health and satisfactory achievement of occupations. The model categorises and sub-divides occupations and the environment as well as the individual skills an individual needs to carry out occupations as follows:

- *Occupations (Self-maintenance, productivity and leisure)*: They describe individuals as categorising the same occupation in different ways and it being important to ascertain the *individual's* opinion of the occupation's categorisation. They (Reed and Sanderson 1999) clearly maintain that it is important for the individual to have a balance of self maintenance, productivity and leisure in their occupations, but that it is up to the individual to determine the nature of that balance. Their description of productivity as more than work means that it could be applicable to the roles any individual (whether a worker or not) engages in when regarding themself as contributing something, whether to family, friends or society.

- *Environment (the physical environment (inorganic), the psychobiological (organic) environment and the societal-cultural environment)*: Reed and Sanderson (1999) see the environments as having two influences on the individual's ability to perform occupations. One is positive, where the environment is one that facilitates and encourages the occupation, whilst the other is negative, where the environment is one that hinders and obstructs the occupation. One could, therefore, see the occupational therapist's role as one of primarily promoting a facilitating environment for clients to carry out occupations within.
- *Skills:* These were initially (1983) divided into the familiar areas of motor, sensory, cognitive, intra-personal and inter-personal skills. They were amended in 1992 and 1999 and ultimately described as sensorimotor components, cognitive integration and cognitive components and psychosocial skills and psychological components.

The trouble with this model (or it may be its strength) is that Reed and Sanderson (1992) never really felt that models actually provide direction for practice, but that the role of a model is one of 'organising the concepts that address a group of problems' (p. 53). Therefore, any suggestions for the model's practical application are purely subjective and could easily be interpreted differently.

## Model of Human Occupation (originally 1985)

Kielhofner and Burke (1980) recognised a need for occupational therapy to have a more generic model or framework to work with than was in use at the time. Building on the work of Mary Reilly, they felt that occupational therapy practice was facing a dilemma, which was leading to fragmentation of the profession, due to the non-existence of a universal guiding structure. They put forward the hypothesis that the development of one model of practice, which could be used by all occupational therapists, would prevent the profession from competing with itself via the range of interventions being used and consequently lead to the growth and development of occupational therapy practice and theory. This led to the Model of Human Occupation as published by Kielhofner in 1985, which provided occupational therapists with a formalised guiding structure for both practice and research. The model uses systems theory heavily and feels that it is essential that in order to achieve the goal of occupational therapy – independence for individuals – it is necessary that the make-up of the individual is fully understood. It states clearly that occupational therapists should not concern themselves with separate parts of the human being but consider the person as a total entity, that is the sum of all the parts. In order to be able to do this, an understanding of all aspects of the individual and their environment is required. The model is built on the following assumptions:

- Each person is an *open system*, that is we receive energy and information and use all parts of the system together in order to interpret and organise this and produce a consequential behaviour or action.
- Each person is an *occupational being*, that is we have an inbuilt urge to explore and master environments through the occupations we carry out. These *occupations* are categorised as *self-care, leisure, work and rest* and have a distinct effect on our lifestyle.
- The *physical and social environment* in which we live influence our behaviour and actions via a number of different layers such as *objects, tasks, social groups and culture*, which act as the feedback to our occupational performance.

The Model of Human Occupation offers an explanation of how behaviour is organised by the individual. It attempts to define the *throughput* area of the open system, that is how intake is translated to output via the subsystems within the individual.

In the initial description of the model, Kielhofner (1985) proposed that this internal interpretation and organisation of information took place in a hierarchical structure of sub-systems as follows:

- Volition
- Habituation
- Performance

In later versions of the model (Kielhofner 1995, 2002, 2008), this hierarchy was transformed into what was described as a heterarchy, wherein the order in which the sub-systems were considered or used in practice was determined by the importance that the person engaging in occupations, or the therapist attributed to it. In all versions of the model the *volition* sub-system is composed of an individual's personal views, feelings and attitudes towards their own abilities, desires and fears. It is through volition that individuals choose and develop their daily occupations and thus gain control or mastery over their environment. The *habituation* sub-system is responsible for organising behaviours and actions. It allows the individual to carry out complex actions and patterns of behaviour in a manner that often becomes automatic. It involves the identification of personal roles and is also responsible for arranging elements of behaviour into routines and in developing these routines into habits, thus providing a structure and consistency to everyday actions. The *performance* or in later versions of the model, the mind-brain-body performance sub-system produces the actions of the individual to allow for occupational behaviours. It provides the end product of the throughput element of the open-system, that is output. It includes the individual's perception of the need for action, the ability to problem solve and take appropriate decisions and the production of the required movement or action. This is influenced by the level of order or disorder within the individual's ability to maintain and carry out occupations, which is in turn influenced by illness or disability.

## The Canadian Model of Occupational Performance (Townsend et al 1997, 2002) and the CMOP-E (Townsend and Polatjko 2007)

The Canadian Model of Occupational Performance (now CMOP-E) evolved from a nationally recognised need to determine ways of ensuring the quality of consistency of service delivery by health care professionals in Canada. Its intention is to demonstrate the way in which the theory of occupational therapy is embedded within enabling occupation in its clients. It builds upon the work of Mosey (1980), Reed and Sanderson (1980), Kielhofner and Burke (1980) and Canada's own Guidelines for Client-Centred Practice. The model places greater emphasis on the individual as a spiritual being than do the previously discussed models and in its more recent metamorphosis (Townsend and Polatjko 2007) clearly identifies itself with occupational science. It requires occupational therapists to consider individuals as a complex system made up of mind, body and spirituality, with spirituality being seen as the core of the individual. The CMOP-E utilises the theories of many disciplines such as anthropology, education, economics, management, medicine and sociology in order to develop a unique, synthesis of knowledge that enables an understanding of occupation and its relationship to health. Whilst individual components of the theoretical knowledge base may be shared with other professionals, the model feels that it is the links between the components, relating specifically to occupational engagement within a person's environment that identify it as a model of the unique profession of occupational therapy.

The model's main assumptions are as follows:

- People have an innate need to engage in occupation.
- There is a very close relationship between an individual's occupational engagement and their environment.
- Occupation, the person, the environment and spirituality are inter-connected.

This model is based on the belief that all occupational behaviour is derived from the individual's mental, physical, sociocultural and spiritual make-up and skills. When there is a well-balanced, fully integrated combination of these elements within their environment, an individual is able to engage in occupations as a healthy, competent person, whether or not they have an illness or disability.

With the essence of the person or the spirituality of the person taken as read and seen as central, where spirituality is our way of defining ourselves as unique human beings with our own individual belief systems about ourselves, the model is made up of three interacting elements:

- *Performance and engagement*: Three categories of occupational engagement and performance are identified, but it should be recognised that the nature of occupational performance will change as individuals develop as will the balance of occupations required for healthy, functional living. The model views it as essential to see these categories from the perspective of the client not the therapist. Like the other models discussed in the preceding text, the categories have changed over the years of the model's development, but currently they are categorised as *cognitive* (intellectual ability, memory, comprehension perceptions reasoning), *affective, social* and *emotional functions or skills*, including intra- and inter-personal abilities) and *physical* (all sensory motor functions) aspects of the person's ability to engage in occupations.

- *Occupation*: The three areas of occupation are categorised as *self-care, productivity and leisure* in a similar way to Reed and Sanderson (1983).
- *Environment*: There are four environmental components and these are as follows:
  1. *Cultural* (ethnicity and routine practices of particular social groups)
  2. *Institutional* (organisational policies, governmental policies legal services and economic issues; this area of environment probably affects the therapist as much as it affects the client)
  3. *Physical* (both natural and man-made surroundings that are concrete and inorganic)
  4. *Social* (relationships, social groupings)

The section Models of Occupational Therapy has outlined the theories that I view to be the current models of occupational therapy devised by and utilised within our profession. It does not include an overview of some theories that other occupational therapists might regard as models. That is, because I do not view those other theories as our profession's models, but as something else; philosophy, approaches or even simply ways of working (such as the problem-solving process often called the occupational therapy process). These other theories (particularly approaches) can of course be *used* by us as occupational therapists, but become dangerous to our professional identity if *used to define* our profession.

## Use of the models in occupational therapy

Each of the three models (as defined in this chapter) outlined in the preceding text offers models for occupational therapists to use in any workplace setting. As such they provide a structural framework for occupational therapists to organise their practice. They do not provide a prescription for action, rather a set of guides to enable us to ensure that we can work to the full extent of our professional expertise, and thus provide the client with an intervention that meets their occupational needs. They are frameworks that assist us to clearly identify areas and causes of occupational interruption, and provide efficient and effective intervention plans that focus on occupational interruption and not just symptoms. They are, therefore, *models for* not *models of* occupational therapy (see Chapter 2). By the clear identification of issues such as volition, psychobiological environment and identifying the spirituality of the client, occupational therapy planning and intervention remains client centred. The models require therapists to recognise the importance of therapist/client interactions in order to gain a full picture of the complex human being and the comprehensive understanding of their occupational behaviour. They all also ensure that therapists are aware of the influences of the environment on occupational performance. Thus, the aim of occupational therapy should be to provide an environment that enables an individual to attain his or her maximum occupational potential and thus enhance self-worth.

# Conclusion

This chapter has offered my definitions of theory terms within occupational therapy that are used throughout this book. These terms and their inter-relationships have been tried and tested in a number of practice settings with which I have worked. They have offered therapists in those settings a clear structure within which to base their use of the occupational therapy specific theory included within profession specific models. Commonly used profession-specific models have been outlined and placed within the wider historical context of the gradual development of occupational therapy theory. The reader is directed to the model-specific literature identified in the Further reading section at the end of this chapter for more in-depth description of the specific models. This chapter intended to offer term definition and overviews of models that the practitioners writing about their use of models in subsequent chapters of this book allude to rather than a full description of the models themselves.

In conclusion to this chapter, I suggest that with all models, which expand the holistic philosophy of occupational therapy, it is important to consider *all* the areas outlined in the models, even if a client seems to have no obvious problem in that area; or the workplace of the therapist does not address issues in that area. Using models in this manner ensures a level of occupational therapy investigation that is truly holistic and prevents us from viewing ourselves as a physical, paediatric or mental health occupational therapist (to name but a few), but as an occupational therapist. It also avoids the trap of basing occupational therapy practice in approaches to intervention (which are generic to all professions) rather than occupation and occupational therapy based theory.

# References

Brint, S. (1993) Eliot Friedson's contribution to the sociology of professions. *Work and Occupations* 20(3), 259–278.

Canadian Association of Occupational Therapy (CAOT) (1986, 1987, 1991) *Occupational Therapy Guidelines for Client Centred Practice*. Toronto: CAOT Publications.

Cole, M.B. and Tuffano, R. (2008) *Applied Theories in Occupational Therapy: A Practical Approach*. Thorofare, NJ: Slack Inc.

Creek, J. (2003) *Occupational Therapy Defined as a Complex Intervention*. London: College of Occupational Therapists.

Duncan, A.S. (ed.) (2006) *Foundations for Practice in Occupational Therapy*, 4th edn. Edinburgh: Elsevier Churchill Livingstone.

Fidler, G.S. and Fidler, J.W. (1963) *Occupational Therapy: A Communication Process in Psychiatry*. New York: Macmillan.

Hagedorn, R. (1992) *Occupational Therapy: Foundations for Practice, Models, Frames of Reference and Core Skills*. London: Churchill Livingstone.

Hagedorn, R. (2001) *Foundations for Practice in Occupational Therapy*. Edinburgh: Churchill Livingstone.

Health Professions Council (2007) *Standards of Proficiency Occupational Therapists.* United Kingdom: Health Professions Council.

Health Professions Council (2009) *Standards of Education and Training.* United Kingdom: Health Professions Council.

Hugman, R. (1991) *Power in the Caring Professions.* Basingstoke: Macmillan Education.

Iwama, M.K. (2006) *The Kawa Model: Culturally Relevant Occupational Therapy.* Philadelphia: Churchill Livingstone.

Jacobs, K. and Jacobs, L. (2009) *Quick Reference Dictionary for Occupational Therapy.* Thorofare, NJ: Slack.

Kielhofner, G. (1985) *A Model of Human Occupation.* Baltimore: Lippincott, Williams and Wilkins.

Kielhofner, G. (1995) *A Model of Human Occupation*, 2nd edn. Baltimore: Lippincott, Williams and Wilkins.

Kielhofner, G. (2002) *A Model of Human Occupation*, 3rd edn. Baltimore: Lippincott, Williams and Wilkins.

Kielhofner, G. (2008) *A Model of Human Occupation*, 4th edn. Baltimore: Lippincott, Williams and Wilkins.

Kielhofner, G. and Burke, J. (1980) A model of human occupation, Part I: conceptual framework and content. *American Journal of Occupational Therapy* 34, 572–581.

Kielhofner, G. and Forsyth, K. (2006) Activity Analysis in Duncan A.S. Skills for Practice in Occupational Therapy, pp. 91–103. Oxford: Churchill Livinsgtone Elsevier.

Kuhn, T. (1996) *The Structure of Scientific Revolutions*, 3rd edn. London: University of Chicago Press.

Law, M., Cooper, B., Strong, S., Stewart, D., Rigby, P. and Letts, L. (1996) The Person-Environment-Occupation Model: a transactive approach to occupational performance. *Canadian Journal of Occupational Therapy* 63(1), 9–23.

Mosey, A.C. (1968) Recapitulation of ontogenesis: a theory for the practice of occupational therapy. *American Journal of Occupational Therapy* 22(5), 426–438.

Mosey, A.C. (1974) An alternative: the Biopsychosocial Model. *American Journal of Occupational Therapy March* 28(3), 137–140.

Mosey, A.C. (1980) A Model for Occupational Therapy. *Occupational Therapy in Mental Health Spring* 1, 11–31.

Mosey, A.C. (1981) *Occupational Therapy: Configuration of a Profession.* New York: Raven Press.

Mosey, A.C. (1986) *Psychosocial Components of Occupational Therapy.* New York: Raven Press.

Reed, K.L. (1984) *Models of Practice in Occupational Therapy.* Baltimore: Lippincott, Williams and Wilkins.

Reed, K.L. and Sanderson, S.N. (1983) *Concepts of Occupational Therapy*, 2nd edn. Baltimore: Lippincott, Williams and Wilkins.

Reed, K.L. and Sanderson, S.N. (1992) *Concepts of Occupational Therapy*, 3rd edn. Baltimore: Lippincott, Williams and Wilkins.

Reed, K.L. and Sanderson, S.N. (1999) *Concepts of Occupational Therapy*, 4th edn. Baltimore: Lippincott, Williams and Wilkins.

Reilly, M. (1962) Occupational Therapy Can Be One of The Great Ideas of 20th Century Medicine. *American Journal of Occupational Therapy* XVI(1), 87–105.

Smith, R. (1992) Theory: an entitlement to understanding. *Cambridge Journal of Education* 22(3), 387–398.

Townsend, E., Stanton, S., Law, M., Polatajko, H., Baptiste, S., Thompson-Franson, T., Kramer, C., Swedlove, F., Brintnell, S. and Campanile, L. (1997) *Enabling Occupation: An Occupational Therapy Perspective*. Ottawa, ON: CAOT ACE.

Townsend, E., Stanton, S., Law, M., Polatajko, H., Baptiste, S., Thompson-Franson, T., Kramer, C., Swedlove, F., Brintnell, S. and Campanile, L. (2002) *Enabling Occupation: An Occupational Therapy Perspective*. Ottawa, ON: CAOT ACE.

Townsend, E.A. and Polatajko, H.J. (2007). *Enabling Occupation II: Advancing an Occupational Therapy Vision for Health, Well-being & Justice through Occupation*. Ottawa, ON: CAOT ACE.

Tyrer, P. and Steinberg, D. (2005) *Models for Mental Disorder Chichester*. Chichester: John Wiley & Sons.

Turpin, M. and Iwama, M.K. (2011) *Using Occupational Therapy Models in Practice*. Edinburgh: Elsevier Churchill Livingstone.

Witz, A. (1992) *Professions and Patriarchy*. New York: Routledge.

## Further reading

Kielhofner, G. (2008) *A Model of Human Occupation*, 4th edn. Baltimore: Lippincott, Williams and Wilkins.

Reed, K.L. and Sanderson, S.N. (1999) *Concepts of Occupational Therapy*, 4th edn. Baltimore: Lippincott, Williams and Wilkins.

Townsend, E.A. and Polatajko, H.J. (2007). *Enabling Occupation II: Advancing an Occupational Therapy Vision for Health, Well-being & Justice through Occupation*. Ottawa, ON: CAOT ACE.

## Chapter 4

# From *Strands* to *The Invisibles*: from a technical to a moral mode of reflective practice

*Della Fish*

---

**Key points**

- Models of reflection
- A journey through models of reflection
- Strands of reflection
- The invisibles of reflective professional practice

---

Progress in virtue is not just a matter of behaving differently – more steadfastly or resolutely, ... but of becoming perceptively and affectively attuned to moral aspects of experience that the less morally virtuous cannot even discern. It is a matter of personal change or development on the part of agents, not just of behaviour modification or increase in intellectual knowledge ...

Carr (2004) (In Dunne and Hogan)

## Introduction

This chapter traces the emergence of two different resources to aid reflection that I have developed (with colleagues) for health care practitioners during the last 22 years. The first of these two resources has had some influence within occupational therapy and other health care professions for several decades, but without, I think, achieving much change in the focus of professionals, about who they are or might become as practitioners. The second resource is already proving to be of greater benefit to a wide range of health care practitioners, being more robust in its critique of current times, offering greater insight into what really drives practice and enabling practitioners to begin to see *the person* they can become. I am grateful for this opportunity to alert occupational therapist readers to these new ideas.

---

*Using Occupational Therapy Theory in Practice*, First Edition. Edited by Gail Boniface and Alison Seymour.
© 2012 Blackwell Publishing Ltd. Published 2012 by Blackwell Publishing Ltd.

I developed the resource, known as 'Strands of Reflection', with Sheila Twinn in the late 1980s (Fish et al 1989, 1991). It delineated four aspects (or strands) of an event that we argued needed to be reflected on to ensure the emergence from that practice of deeper understanding. By and large, what *Strands* sought to achieve was a greater understanding about the clinical event itself. It did attempt to nudge the focus of the practitioner's reflection from the technical rational to the professional artistry elements of the clinician's work and (in the third strand) it did ask questions about the person the practitioner was, but it did not really succeed in highlighting this. Mainly, it drew attention to the characteristics of the particular piece of practice itself. Further, the artistry that *Strands* sought to illuminate was partly obscured by the technical rational view of practice that ran like an avalanche through the last two decades of the twentieth century, such that by the 1990s any other view of practice had been virtually wiped out.

More recently, during the first decade of the twenty-first century, again in critical response to the technical rationalism now so smothering a professional discourse, that it has become the unquestioned norm, I have developed with my colleague Linda de Cossart, a set of educational resources called *The Invisibles*. By contrast to *Strands*, these are designed to promote rigorous reflection by the doctor/surgeon/health care practitioner about their personal mode of practice in respect of a particular event or case in their own practice. That is, *The Invisibles* focuses on and asks questions about the soundness and the wisdom of the practitioner's thinking processes and their judgements in respect of a specific patient case, or a clinical process (de Cossart and Fish 2005; Fish and de Cossart 2007). Thus, this time, the entire resource is concerned at least as much with ontology (the person the practitioner is and how they understand and express their moral and clinical responsibilities) as with epistemology (the nature of professional knowledge drawn upon) and the technicalities of patient care. That is, *The Invisibles* provide resources designed to oppose the technical mode of practice with the moral mode and are more appropriate for practitioners who seriously seek to move on from the technical rationality of the Twentieth Century! (see later and also in Carr (2004) in Dunne and Hogan).

Thus, this chapter contains a story here with a moral. A story concerning the use of strands of reflection and of how, without frequent critical review by individual professionals and professions themselves, an idea made concrete as a resource for use in education at a particular time can continue to influence professional practice even after the context has changed, the resource has become inadvertently distorted and uncomfortable, and has in fact been replaced as outmoded by its creator!

## The development of *Strands*

### An overview

*Strands* was developed as a model for use by those who were learning to become practitioners, to enable them to learn from and through their practice. It was a creature of its time, being shaped by the context of the late 1980s, when Schön's (1987) *Educating the reflective practitioner* had only just been published and ideas about how to support serious reflective processes in health care and teaching were in their infancy. *Strands* was designed for use by supervisors with their pre-service practitioners. This resource has several characteristics that have re-emerged with greater emphasis in the more recent *Invisibles*. Its gradual distortion was partly an inevitable result of a *Chinese whispers* approach to spreading its influence in the professions, and partly because what was intended to be a set of ideas for informed supervisors to use *with* supervisees, became an *instrument* used by practitioners more generally. As a result, although *Strands* was intended as model, it was also described as a set of guidelines and certainly was not intended to offer the rigidity that developed inadvertently around its ideas, as some enthusiastic teachers and practitioners began to impose it on learners. This may have been because it was a very early example in the literature of a systematic approach to reflection. Certainly it was because *Strands* was born into a world in which health care education was besotted by *models as rigid structures for action.*

As has already been outlined in Chapter 2, the problem with models, of course, is that if used indiscriminately, they can both rigidify processes and become reductionist. Thus, what was intended as a set of four strands to be used to guide those seeking to learn from pre-service practice alongside a more knowledgeable senior became (particularly in occupational therapy) a concrete model for all who wished to show that they were serious practitioners in their own individual practice. For this larger purpose, it was often reduced to the more comfortable first, second and fourth strands (leaving out the third and more challenging one). It thus became something it never set out to be!

To understand *Strands*, it is important to recognise that it offered a set of four intertwining aspects or threads of practice, which when considered together, we argued, would enable us to make deeper sense of something that had happened in our practice. These threads were as follows:

1. The Factual strand (recounting the facts of the event)
2. The Retrospective strand (identifying the key patterns that emerged in the event)
3. The Sub-stratum strand ('uncovering and exploring critically the personal theory that underlies the piece of practice')
4. The Connective strand (considering how present theory and practice might relate to future theory and practice)

This last strand carried a warning that all practice events are unique and that applying directly what has been learnt in one situation to a new one is never possible. We also suggested that the *significant event* to be reflected on should be a serious learning opportunity that was worth exploring further, rather than for use with those negative experiences usually referred to as *critical clinical incidents*. Thus, we encouraged reflecting on positive as well as negative aspects of practice.

### How strands came about

*Strands* arose from a small piece of research I conducted with Sheila Twinn and our research assistant, Bridget Purr, on what supervisors of pre-service practice in teaching and in Health Visiting did to enable their supervisees to learn from their time in practice.

We chose these two professions because they represented two very different courses of professional preparation, for which we ourselves had responsibility (the teaching course under scrutiny being an undergraduate course, the Health Visiting one being postgraduate).

This research, called the HELPP project that stood for 'How to Enable students to Learn through Professional Practice', sprang from the early days of introducing reflection in teaching and health care as a serious means of 'turning experience into learning', to quote the title of an iconic book of the period (Boud et al 1985). Our stated intention was:

> NOT [*sic*] to offer the definitive framework for shaping and interpreting practice but to provide one starting point as a means of focusing discussion, investigation, reflection, analysis and theorising about the supervision of practice and how student's learning might best be fostered.
>
> (Fish et al 1989, p. x)

The approach to reflection then in vogue was that of providing the learner with a very specific series of key questions or ideas to use to ensure that the process of recapturing and reviewing a practice event was rigorous and that it would yield up important truths about working within a profession.

The data reported in Fish et al (1989) showed that the supervisors we observed in the two professional preparation courses we targeted were not in fact very adept at quickly pulling out of an observed event of practice the key learning issues, and certainly were not enabling their learners to pinpoint such issues for themselves, let alone facilitating critical thinking about them. *Strands* was developed in our second publication, as our response to this. That is, it was prompted by the needs of practice, and we articulated clearly (Fish et al 1991, pp. 12–14) that in here, 'it was also a response to what we saw as the overly technical rational view of practice developing nationally'. We did not know at that time just how far the technical rational view would take over the whole world of professional practice! Our response to this, using Schön's work (1983, 1987), was to try to lay bare and celebrate the artistry of practice (hence the emphasis on professional judgement).

We were, naturally, duly pleased to learn that *Strands* was being taken up by a number of health care professions at the time, including occupational therapy, physiotherapy, nursing and health visiting. This is likely to have been because, in the early 1990s, there were very few other supports in this area. Those that did exist were either very broad, like Gibbs' famous model (Gibbs 1988) that, though it does take the practitioner's feelings into account, asks questions that are very broad and do not invite detailed criticality; or like the early work of Johns (Johns 1994), which formed a rather inflexible protocol offering some factual questions but not leading to any probing or critical thinking about what emerged. By comparison, we offered questions that sought to engage the practitioner in deeper thinking within each of our four strands. But these questions were only meant as examples of the kinds of things to consider within each section. They were not there to be answered as a routine, although that is how they were treated (which is also much as how John's questions are treated).

In Fish et al (1989, 1991), we made the important but unrecognised point that the guidance offered arose from a small piece of research that focused on the *practice* of supervisors as teachers helping learners to reflect on their pre-service practice. The first publication reported that the supervisor or supervisee interaction (after the observed event) shared broadly the same characteristics across both professions (even though one was undergraduate and one postgraduate in nature). More interestingly, eleven clear points emerged from the transcripts of those interactions about 'how supervisors fostered learning through practice via reflection'. These points were listed as follows:

- Being alert to the varied characteristics of the placement.
- Being aware of the range of possibilities for action.
- Drawing upon previous relevant experience.
- Having in mind previously formulated personal theory.
- Drawing upon knowledge of relevant formal theory.
- Taking account of personal values.
- Being aware of how these relate to professional frames of reference.
- Being able to make professional judgements.
- Being able to act upon a decision.
- Continually evaluating a decision and its effects.
- Recognising that professional artistry lies in the alchemy of the combination of the above categories on each unique occasion.

(Fish et al 1989, p. 36)

In those days it was common, following Schön (1983, 1987) to oppose the technical rational view of professional practice with professional artistry! But, in preparing this chapter I have been astonished in revisiting this work, which I have not re-read for many years, to see just how many of the ideas listed above I seem to have taken up in detail during the rest of my working life, and how many of them, even then, were aimed at promoting a moral mode of practice as opposed to a technical one.

## The technical and the moral modes of practice

Since these terms enshrine ideas that are at the heart of this chapter, I offer the following definitions of them, as used here.

When professionals practice in the *technical mode*, they engage in seeing practice as an episodic activity involving a set of skills or competencies that, alongside attitudes and knowledge, are said to constitute the total sum of professional practice 'such that anyone with half a brain and no special training might do it' (Carr 2004, p. 108). Thus *good practice* is seen as exhibited by those who behave as skilled practitioners who are also appropriately knowledgeable, and who apply general principles to practical problems as if simply obeying rules automatically makes them a moral practitioner. This casts professionals into the role of technician and construes professional effectiveness 'largely in terms of the cultivation of a range of performatively measurable skills' (Carr 2004, p. 108). Such practitioners are in fact not in control of their own practice but merely agents of practice as set down by others. They are obedient to convention and do not engage in critiquing it. Neither do they see that part of the development of their practice is about developing themselves. This kind of mindset means that the reflection that they carry out on their own practice, and any developments they engage in, are shaped by a mindset that often ignores reflective prompts that drive for critique of current convention.

By contrast, the *moral mode* of practice (as first described by Aristotle) is at least as much about the kind of person one is, as it is about the skills, and knowledge one has. Here, the practitioner is their own agent and their very choice of strategies and skills is derived from knowledge of a range of possibilities available and a careful selection of these to suit the particular moral purpose. Thus the practitioner working in the moral mode of practice seeks what is best for their patient or client, at all costs, including even their own best interests. Here the practitioner's moral responses to a piece of practice draws them to reflect in ways that:

> aim as far as possible to get to the bottom of things, and [they see] getting to the bottom of things is above all a matter of making *myself* more honest, courageous, self-controlled, just, caring and so on for other human virtues.
>
> (Carr 2004, p. 107)

Here, good practice is not about personal gain, but about aspiring to do the morally right thing and trying to acquire these virtues, through submitting to a moral authority that transcends a personal or social agenda (aspiring to truth that lies beyond any and all sectional interests). In the end, such virtue becomes its own reward (Carr 2004).

If, as I have already outlined, *Strands* did not, for a variety of reasons, engage professionals to reflect at the deeper level and to work towards a more moral mode of practice, how far does *The Invisibles* (Fish and de Cossart 2007) fair in this enterprise?

## The development of *The Invisibles*

### How The Invisibles came about

In 1998, the focus of my work shifted to the education of postgraduate doctors and surgeons. This firstly involved providing advice on teaching to hospital consultants of all specialties whose role (and contract) includes teaching their juniors in the clinical setting until those juniors complete their Specialty Training and are ready to apply for consultant posts. In some specialties, this is a period of about 12 years from entering practice; in some, it is 9 or so. Later, in 2002, I worked with The Royal College of Surgeons to develop the first formal curriculum for postgraduate doctors in their early years of training. As a result, I was caught up in what was called Modernising Medical Careers, and that imposed on medicine and surgery what in my opinion were a very poorly drafted set of curricula, based largely on the propositional knowledge, and the observable and measurable elements of practice. More recently (since 2005), I have been involved across three deaneries in enabling medical and surgical consultants to become more advanced teachers by means of Masters Pathways in Teaching and Learning in the clinical setting. For most consultants, this has constituted the first formal education for teaching they will have experienced.

By contrast to *Strands* (which was a theoretical response to a practical problem that emerged from researching practice) *The Invisibles*, which I created 24 years later, was a practical response to a theoretical problem. This resource emerged as a result of discontent with a national curriculum imposed from above on postgraduate medical education. The technical rational world having moved on to envelop almost all thinking about professional practice, this curriculum was concerned *only* with those aspects of medical and surgical practices that could be observed and measured. Frustration that the invisible elements of practice were so undervalued (or barely recognised), coupled with awareness that the curriculum had not been properly developed from a full analysis of practice (see Fish and Coles 2005), led us to develop a research project designed to unearth and explore those invisible but vital elements that actually drive medical, surgical and health care practice. This involved my working very closely over a long period with a very senior practitioner (Linda de Cossart), theorising her practice (de Cossart and Fish 2005), and then checking the outcomes of this against the practice of a range of doctors, surgeons and health care practitioners. The results of this understanding we then shaped into educational resources designed to enable all health care practitioners to explore their practice in depth (Fish and de Cossart 2007).

Thus, *The Invisibles* arose from a 4-year research programme in which firstly Linda as a clinician and I as an educator worked together in attempting to make as much detailed sense of her daily practice as possible (see Fish 2009). In exploring the invisible drivers of her practice, we worked to make explicit in words or diagrams both the implicit and the 'top end' of the tacit elements of her work. We recognised that some of our tacit knowing and thinking is so deep that it is not recoverable, and some is so difficult to explicate that it is ineffable, thus making it expressible only in figurative language. We then worked to find ways of conceptualising as many invisible elements of practice as possible. We later worked to turn our concepts into educational resources and to explain how they might be used in the practice setting to respond to a range of learning opportunities. We also indicated how these opportunities might be identified. The next section offers an overview of *The Invisibles*.

### An overview of The Invisibles

A great strength of the work on *The Invisibles* was that it was shared between an educator and an eminent surgeon. Between us we found a common way of understanding firstly the deeper characteristics of professional practice as enacted by a practitioner recognised widely as a wise clinician. Secondly, we elucidated the educational requirements of clinical practice by hewing out of our two different languages a congenial means of conveying these ideas that was intelligible to us both. As I expressed it later in a more detailed exploration of our work: 'we may have contributed to a new turn in the discourse of medical education' (Fish, 2009, p.149).

We also took account of the fact that times had changed ideas about reflection and its role in learning and professional development. There is now more criticality about models and protocols. Guidelines are more acceptable, are recognised as more flexible and are seen as a support rather than a straightjacket. Further, there is far more interest in and far more understanding of *professional judgement*. One contribution to this, along the way to *The Invisibles*, was Fish and Coles (eds) (1998), *Developing Professional Judgement in the Heath Care Professions*. This was a collection of chapters by a wide range of health practitioners, all of them examining their professional judgements in a particular case.

*The Invisibles* offers a set of educational resources designed to help postgraduate practitioners to explore in depth a case, or a procedure, or a simulation, or a significant event in their practice. (In what follows, I shall use the term 'case' to stand for a particular piece of practice.) In enabling the practitioner, in respect of a particular case or event, to explore in detail themselves and the drivers of their own practice, they are a development of the third (and often ignored) thread of *Strands*, called the *sub-stratum strand*.

Eight invisible elements emerged during our research (none of them required in any detail by any of the formal medical curricula).

These involve practitioners who explore a specific piece of practice in:

- recognising the significance of the contextual clues (including the influence of the person the practitioner is at that time) and digging down into how they influence the way that piece of practice is understood;
- considering their professionalism in the case;
- revealing the range of knowledge they have drawn on during the case;
- laying bare their thinking processes;
- pinpointing and critiquing their professional judgements;
- seeing beyond the immediacy of the case details;
- using all of these means of exploration in the service of the patient, by exploring the quality of the therapeutic relationship that they establish with the patient; and
- widening the view of the issues involved in the case and thus seeing it anew.

For each of these eight elements, we invented icons that work as heuristics (reminders of the central idea of that element). These can be found at www.ED4MEDPRAC.co.uk. We also offered an explanation of each idea and a set of prompts to help the practitioner to produce both oral and written reflection on the case under scrutiny.

## From talking to clinical reflective writing

Talking is the first natural means of reflecting, and the case being explored needs to be presented to a senior by a learning practitioner through a professional conversation where the senior listens carefully and then aids a deeper exploration. But what is the case being explored? It is useful to remember that for every patient case there exists a case of the learning practitioner who is responsible for the patient. Thus, the reflective conversation about the case should not only seek to explore the patient case experience but also the learner's view of that experience and their consequential learning derived from that exploration.

What we have come to call 'Clinical Reflective Writing', should then follow. A good starting point is a set of bullet points that can firstly be linked up into a simple paragraph and then be gradually turned into a piece of clinical reflective writing that fleshes out the case in detail prompted by the eight heuristics. As we pointed out in Fish and Coles (1998), the learning is actually *in the writing.* That is, the process of writing is what enables the learning. This is not a matter of thinking it all out and then setting down the resulting understanding in writing afterwards. Rather, the learning and understanding emerge during and from the writing. In encouraging practitioners to engage with this writing, we invented what we have come to call a 'rainbow draft', in which the details prompted by each of the invisibles is introduced in a particular coloured type face into the original paragraph of black prose that itself contains just a brief narrative of the case. An example is to be found on www.ED4MEDPRAC.co.uk.

It is not necessary to write in detail about all eight elements, and certainly not in a *one off* piece of writing. Rather, the idea is to tackle whichever of these elements seems to need deeper understanding by the particular learning practitioner (prompted perhaps, if they are junior doctors or surgeons by the particular requirements of the Foundation or specialty curriculum through which they are learning). This writing needs sympathetic and serious response by the senior colleague/supervisor. Comments in the margin and at the end, with a date and a signature, will validate the writing as worth placing in the learning or appraisal portfolio. Further writing in response to another *invisible* in another colour would further enrich the understanding of that case. This is useful where learners have fewer cases to learn from than in the past. By this means, it is possible to build up a very deep understanding of two or three cases across a 3- or 4-month attachment, by progressively attending to each of the elements in these selected pieces of practice. This can be done in virtually any order, depending on the needs of the practitioner.

Details of how to use clinical reflective writing can be found at the following address http://www.ed4medprac.co.uk/papers.htm. For full details of how to use the invisibles for clinical reflective writing, with examples from senior teachers and their learners see de Cossart and Fish (2011).

## Conclusion

It is the profound hope of Linda de Cossart and myself that *The Invisibles* will be useful for all clinical practitioners seeking to improve their practice by understanding it better. We hope to see the resource used as part of an advanced approach to teaching, which we know medical and surgical consultants are already taking on.

I believe that traditional teaching in health care – in the classroom or the clinical setting – often reinforces, in error, the technical mode of practice in both clinical work and teaching. It does this whenever it consists of little more than 'presenting or providing new knowledge, training in specific job-skills and procedures and encouraging [superficial] reflection on immediate experience' (Fish and Brigley 2010, p. 113). This can lead the learner to be inactive and bored, and certainly does not attend to developing their creative, critical and imaginative abilities. Neither does it respond with sophistication to the complexity and uncertainty of clinical practice. Enhanced teaching, by contrast is based on 'in-depth educational understanding, which, in turn, arises from teachers' exploration of their own clinical and educational values and which attends to and seeks to develop the learner's understanding and values' (Fish and Brigley 2010, p. 114).

By comparison with the traditional (*instrumentalist*) view of teaching as equipping the workforce to do their job, *enhanced* teaching rests on a deeper understanding of the nature of education as emancipatory. This brings with it the moral duty for professionals to be aware of the values (personal and professional) that drive their judgements and actions. It also involves helping learners to consider in detail their clinical judgements and to probe the thinking that leads to them or underpins them.

I hope that *The Invisibles* can, over the next few years, show the impoverished mindset endemic in the technical mode of practice in health care and make some contribution to a greater recognition of the importance of the moral mode of practice. After all, Aristotle knew a thing or two in first drawing our attention to both modes.

## References

Boud, D., Keough, R. and Walker, D. (1985) *Turning Experience into Learning*. London: Kogan Page.

Carr, D. (2004) Rival conceptions of practice in education and teaching. In: *Education and Practice: Upholding the Integrity of Teaching and Learning*, eds J. Dunne and P. Hogan. Oxford: Blackwell Publishing Ltd.

de Cossart, L. and Fish, D. (2005) *Cultivating a Thinking Surgeon: New Perspectives on Clinical Teaching, Learning and Assessment*. Shrewsbury: TFM Publications Ltd.

de Cossart, L. and Fish, D. (eds) (2011) *Enhancing Teaching and Learning in Postgraduate Medicine*. London: Royal Society of Medicine.

Fish, D. (2009) Research as a pragmatic practice: unpredictable means, unforeseeable ends (Chapter 9). In: *Understanding and Researching Professional Practice*, ed. B. Green. Rotterdam: Sense Publications.

Fish, D. and Brigley, S. (2010) Exploring the practice of education: towards enhanced teaching in the clinical setting. In: *Education for Future Practice*, eds J. Higgs, D. Fish, I. Goulter, S. Loftus and F Trede. Rotterdam: Sense Publications.

Fish, D. and Coles, C. (1998) *Developing Professional Judgement in Health Care: Learning through the Critical Appreciation of Practice*. Oxford: Butterworth Heinemann.

Fish, D. and Coles, C. (2005) *Medical Education: Developing a Curriculum for Practice*. Maidenhead: Open University Press.

Fish, D. and de Cossart, L. (2007) *Developing the Wise Doctor*. London: Royal Society of Medicine.

Fish, D., Twinn, S. and Purr, B. (1989) *How to Enable Learning through Professional Practice: A Cross Profession Investigation of Pre-service Practice*. London: West London Institute.

Fish, D., Twinn, S., and Purr, B. (1991) *Promoting Reflection: Improving the Supervision of Practice in Health Visiting and Initial Teacher Education*. London: West London Education.

Gibbs, G. (1988) *Learning by Doing: A Guide to Teaching and Learning Methods*. Oxford: Further Education Unit, Oxford Polytechnic.

Johns, C. (1994) Guided reflection. In: *Reflective Practice in Nursing: The Growth of the Professional Practitioner*, eds A. Palmer, S. Burns and C. Bulman. Oxford: Blackwell Scientific publications.

Schön, D.A. (1983) *The Reflective Practitioner*. London: Arena.

Schön, D.A. (1987) *Educating the Reflective Practitioner*. London: Jossey-Bass Publishers.

## Further reading

Fish, D. and de Cossart, L. (2007) *Developing the Wise Doctor*. London: Royal Society of Medicine.

de Cossart, L. and Fish, D. (eds) (2011) *Enhancing Teaching and Learning in Postgraduate Medicine*. London: Royal Society of Medicine.

# Chapter 5

# The use of self in occupational therapy

*Alison Seymour*

---

**Key points**

- The use of self is the way occupational therapists use the interpersonal relationships and interactions with service users to influence the occupational outcome of interventions
- Occupational therapists can use a number of different theories to enhance the use of self
- Use of self impacts positively upon making intervention outcomes occupationally focussed
- The use of self is the fabric of the occupational therapy umbrella, which helps maintain an occupational focus in practice
- Learning how to use self is inherent in reflective practices and should begin early in occupational therapy curricula and continue throughout one's professional career

---

## Introduction

This chapter sets out to present a personal account of how I have used theory to enhance the use of self in my occupational therapy practice. The use of self is not unique to occupational therapy; therefore, the chapter will explore how I have used theory from other disciplines whilst maintaining the centrality of client-centred practice and occupation within my practice. Referring to the analogy of the umbrella of theory in Chapter 3, the use of self can be viewed as the *fabric* that links occupational therapy theory and its use in practice. This fabric represents the way occupational therapists use the interpersonal relationships and interactions between themselves and service users to influence the occupational outcome of interventions.

The ideas for this chapter have developed through my own personal interest in this area of practice through working with people with mental health problems. However, this chapter should prove useful for all practitioners regardless of the setting they work in. As an occupational therapist, the use of self has been one of the most effective

*Using Occupational Therapy Theory in Practice*, First Edition. Edited by Gail Boniface and Alison Seymour.
© 2012 Blackwell Publishing Ltd. Published 2012 by Blackwell Publishing Ltd.

aspects of practice I have utilised but also at times the most demanding. Having become a university educator, I sometimes feel that this aspect of practice can be neglected from a theoretical perspective within students' learning. Somehow students are expected to have or develop these skills without having an understanding of the theory underpinning them. Without understanding how this body of theory can be used within occupational therapy, it can be easy for students and practitioners to move away from the focus of the philosophy of occupational therapy practice and adopt a more counselling or generic therapy role.

This chapter, therefore, aims to:

- explore how the use of self is defined within occupational therapy theory;
- explore examples of the positive use of self and reflect on some of the challenges experienced in my own practice;
- discuss ethical and professional considerations for the effective use of self within occupational therapy; and
- explore how the use of self can be enhanced and maintained in practice.

## Defining the use of self

As is often the case in occupational therapy theory, there are multiple definitions within the literature as to what constitutes the use of self. According to Taylor et al (2009) and Taylor and Melton (2009), terms such as *therapeutic alliance, developing rapport, intentional self* and *therapeutic/conscious use of self* are all used to define the interpersonal skills and processes that constitute the relationship between the client and the occupational therapist.

The term *conscious use of self* was originally created by Anne Cronin Mosey (1981). By this she refers to a planned, deliberate interaction with another person. She differentiates this from developing rapport that she views as only a part of the conscious use of self. Rapport is the process of establishing a comfortable relationship with your client based on respect whereas the conscious use of self is described as a more, deliberate, 'manipulation of one's responses to assist a client' (p. 96). Mosey's view is that the aim of such interactions is seen as promoting growth and development and improving or maintaining function in clients. This conscious use of self involves the occupational therapist being sensitive to his or her personal response to the client, that is 'how does this client make me feel, what am I experiencing?' (p. 97). This evaluation of personal responses helps the occupational therapist understand clients' feelings that may not be openly expressed and, therefore, gives clues as to the direction or interpersonal stance they may take next.

Finlay (2004) suggests that occupational therapy does not merely aim to increase client skills but to elicit inner change in the individual and it is through the therapeutic relationship that this change occurs. She presents the complexity of the therapeutic relationship from four perspectives. Firstly, the evolving relationship that includes engagement in therapy, collaboration and negotiation, followed by the letting go or ending of the therapeutic relationship. Secondly, ten dimensions of relationship skills are suggested that can be helpful in enhancing positive relationships such as communicating empathy and being reflexive and self-aware. Thirdly, the conscious use of self that refers to 'the deliberate use of mind and body' (Finlay 2004, p. 148) is discussed. Finally, she concludes her discussion by focussing on issues regarding power and collaboration in the therapeutic relationship.

More recently, Taylor (2008) has developed a conceptual framework of the use of self for occupational therapy practice that she calls the Intentional Relationship Model (IRM). This framework acknowledges that the central focus of occupational therapy is occupational engagement and aims to guide the therapist in interpersonal practices (use of self), which will maximise a client's occupational performance and enhance positive therapy outcomes. As a psychologist, she acknowledges that the underpinning concepts for the IRM derive from theory in psychotherapy. In her framework, however, she presents the differences between traditional psychotherapy, the primary aims of which are the interpersonal aspects of the therapy, and occupational therapy where the primary concern is with the occupational outcomes of the relationship. Taylor's (2008) framework is structured around three areas of interpersonal capacity: the interpersonal skill base, ability to use a variety of interpersonal styles (modes) and the capacity for interpersonal reasoning. She contends that her framework was developed to provide a more structured approach to enable occupational therapists to use the self more effectively, whilst maintaining the occupational goals of their interventions. It is designed to be used alongside occupational therapy professional models (Taylor and Melton 2009), such as the Model of Human Occupation (Kielhofner 2008).

Duncan (2006) and Finlay (2004) both argue that the use of self and the negotiation of the therapeutic relationship is the biggest and most important skill that the occupational therapist has. As mentioned earlier, much of the theoretical knowledge in this area of practice is *borrowed* from psychology and I make no apologies for that. Most occupational therapy theory in regards to approaches and interventions is shared with other professions, for example the biomechanical approach, sensory integration and the use of cognitive behavioural therapies. Kielhofner (2008), when discussing this issue acknowledges that the Model of Human Occupation (2008) is intended to be used alongside other theoretical frameworks to allow a comprehensive approach to meet service users' needs. What is important is how we use theory to complement and enhance our occupational focus and maintain our unique occupational therapy role. Thus, for much of the rest of this chapter, I intend to share how I have used theory to enhance my use of self throughout my occupational therapy practice.

## Using theory in practice: a personal account

My own experience of learning about the use of self began as a student occupational therapist in the early 1980s. The work of Carl Rogers and the humanistic school of psychology were embedded in the curriculum I studied, and although I did not appreciate this at the time, the group work approach to learning about the use of self and the importance of the therapeutic relationship had a lasting effect on me as an occupational therapist.

Rogers first coined the phrase *client-centred practice* in 1939 (Parker 2006). His work is acknowledged as being at the foundation of client-centred therapy. The central tenets of active listening, understanding the internal world of the individual, acceptance and genuineness in the therapeutic relationship have formed the basis of many psychological therapies and counselling styles (Rogers 1951, 1961). The relevance of his contribution to client-centred practice as developed within occupational therapy is recognised within the literature (Law et al 1995; Parker 2006; Taylor 2008).

My own use of these ideas in practice really developed through working in forensic mental health settings. The background offences of the service users and the environmental constraints of the settings made theoretical concepts such as client-centred practice, positive regard and working in partnership somewhat of a challenge at times. However, this view of the therapeutic relationship was exactly what was required in order to motivate and engage the service users in occupations. I also found it necessary to separate the person from the offences, in order to be able to develop constructive, enabling relationships with the service users whilst maintaining clear, professional and therapeutic boundaries. This stance in no way condoned the offending behaviour, but in fact, I found it enabled me to be able to challenge issues of responsibility more effectively once the therapeutic relationship was established.

Another theory that impacted on my use of self was introduced to me when I was a relatively inexperienced occupational therapist working in community mental health. I was often in a position of having to deal with clients in acute distress within their own homes and I remember feeling ill equipped and anxious that I would say the wrong thing thus making the situation worse. Therefore, I decided to undertake a counselling course as a way of enhancing my skills, particularly in the use of self. The theoretical framework of this counselling approach both influenced and enhanced my practice as an occupational therapist within this setting (Egan 1990). The framework, known as *the skilled helper* fits well with other approaches used within occupational therapy and was developed as either a stand-alone approach for counsellors or as an approach that can be incorporated into other areas of professional practice. It has a pragmatic, problem-solving basis, which encourages clients to tell their story, and develop their own goals and helping strategies through the 'working alliance' (Egan 1990, p. 58). This relationship with the therapist is collaborative, respectful and genuine and encourages clients to assume a sense of self-responsibility and enhances their ability to utilise their own resources. Through this course I developed valuable skills in listening and attending, how to use empathy and effective challenging techniques such as the use of immediacy and paradoxical responses. This interpersonal approach helped me to use myself effectively in the relationship with clients to both support and challenge the interpersonal and emotional demands that arise whilst still maintaining a focus on the client's occupational goals.

# Psychodynamic theory

Both of the previously discussed client-centred theoretical approaches have been invaluable in developing my confidence and effectiveness in the use of self throughout my career. However, the most influential theoretical framework that has impacted on my practice as an occupational therapist, in respect of the use of self, has been psychodynamic theory. As a student I was dismissive of this theory but through experience, training and time, I grew to rely on it. This was both to understand and explain the processes of the therapeutic relationships I developed with clients and the processes of the teams I worked in. Using this theoretical understanding enabled me to use myself in the most effective way when collaborating and facilitating occupational change with clients. It gave me a framework for reflection and supervision that not only focussed my professional development on the skills and outcomes of occupational therapy interventions but also the fabric of the relationships and processes of the use of self used within interventions (this concept of use of self as the fabric of the occupational therapy umbrella is also referred to in Chapter 3).

The use of psychodynamic theory within occupational therapy practice is explored very well by Blair and Daniel (2006) and I make no apology for my enthusiasm for this approach, although it has been criticised as having contributed to a crisis of identity within occupational therapy in the past (Barris et al (1983) cited in Blair and Daniel (2006)). My interest focusses on its value as a framework for understanding and using the self whilst maintaining an occupational focus to my practice; a position clearly advocated as far back as the 1960s (Fidler and Fidler 1963). Through undertaking training in psychoanalytic group work, I was introduced to a range of psychotherapy theories; including those of Bion (1961), Foulkes (1983) and Yalom and Leszcz (2005), which I was then able to use in my interactions with individual clients and in group work. These ideas also impacted on my approach to supervision as I recognised that the more complex the clients' presentations were, the more imperative it was to understand and utilise the interpersonal aspect of the therapeutic relationship.

Concepts from psychodynamic theory that I have found most useful include some of the following.

## *Transference*

Transference is described as 'an unconscious process where a person responds to another in a manner similar to the way he or she responded to a significant person in the past' (Finlay 1993, p. 144). Transference occurs in all therapeutic relationships, regardless of the occupational interruption or setting, but is often not recognised or acknowledged within therapeutic interactions by occupational therapists.

Similarly, counter-transference can occur where the occupational therapist unconsciously complies with and behaves in the manner of the expectation that the client has of the therapist (Fidler and Fidler 1963). For instance, a young male client in his 20s who lived a very chaotic, disorganised lifestyle was referred to me in a community mental health setting. His goals included wanting to return to work, which involved him primarily achieving several pre-vocational goals. My experience of working with him was that he was never able to achieve any of the goals we would set collabora- tively. He would then respond angrily to me if he perceived that any of my feedback or interactions with him were negative or critical in nature. In response to this, because he never achieved any of the planned occupational goals, I found myself slipping into a role where I was actually giving him only negative feedback, albeit in a way that I thought was sensitive and constructive. Through supervision, I was able to unpick that he was responding to me as he had done to his teachers at school, where he achieved very little and received a lot of criticism and negative feedback (transference) and I was in fact responding in the manner he expected me too when he failed to achieve the goals we had set (counter-transference). Using this insight, I was then able to discuss with him the pattern of our interactions, and this allowed us to have an open dialogue about what we were both locked into doing. This improved our relationship and I was then able to challenge his chaotic behaviour more effectively using appropriate humour (Mosey 1986).

### Understanding defence mechanisms

Defence mechanisms are seen as one of the central tenets of psychodynamic theory (Blair and Daniel 2006) and can be described as having a protective function in the unconscious protection of unacceptable thoughts and feelings. Defence mechanisms are needed and used by everyone including you as a therapist. Having an understanding of how you and your clients will exhibit different defences is a useful tool in the use of self in practice. Blair and Daniel (2006) and Bateman et al (2000) both describe a similar range of defence mechanisms and some of the most common ones I have experienced in practice are as follows:

* Projection (the externalisation of unacceptable feelings that are then attributed to others)
* Denial (denying, avoiding or forgetting an unpleasant/traumatic external event)
* Rationalisation (excessive attempts to justify behaviour, that is 'yes, but' responses)
* Regression (reverting back to behaviours normally seen at a younger age, that is dependency behaviours)

It is important to remember that defence mechanisms are normally used uncon- sciously and the client is largely unaware of the source of their origin. Within occu- pational therapy practice I am not suggesting that it is our role to uncover and break down these protective defences but recognising and using this knowledge in our in- teractions with clients can help to develop the quality of the therapeutic relationship and help in understanding the occupational problems that clients may be experiencing. For example, I worked with a young woman who frequently projected the idea that people did not like her. This impacted on her social and working life causing her to be very isolated and lonely and therefore reinforcing the idea that she was not liked. We were able to explore the idea that she was actually projecting her own feelings of low self-esteem onto others as a way of protecting herself from perceived rejection. Through the understanding of this formulation of her difficulties, she was able to explore different ways of interacting with people and trying out new social and leisure activities. Over time, as this cycle of projection was challenged, she began to view herself and others in a better way.

### Setting boundaries

The setting of professional boundaries within the therapeutic relationship is vital for the protection of both yourself and the client. The maintenance of professional behaviour is embedded in COT (2010) and is a requirement for continued registration with the Health Professions Council (HPC 2008) in the United Kingdom. Taylor (2008) presents a very useful discussion of what constitutes professional behaviour within the therapeutic relationship particularly in respect to the use of self within occupational therapy. Maintaining professional boundaries is *always* the responsibility of the occupational therapist and deserves careful consideration throughout practice wherever it occurs (HPC 2008). This aspect of the therapeutic relationship and use of self is one that students and newly registered occupational therapists may find particularly challenging. The nuances and individuality of each unique therapeutic relationship may not be overtly observed and understood and therefore may require explanation and exploration within a supervisory relationship.

Using psychodynamic theory has again helped me to recognise boundary testing with clients, behaviours that are often again unconscious to the clients themselves. Some of the most common boundary testing behaviours that I have experienced include the following:

- Doorknob comments (Taylor 2008): Throw away comments made as a client is leaving, or waiting until the last 5 minutes of a session before disclosing something really important.
- Projection of emotions onto the therapist: Displaying feelings of anger, or inappropriate humour to cover up other emotions.
- Attempting to change the nature of the therapeutic relationship: Through trying to give gifts, wanting self-disclosure about your life and experiences.
- Sabotaging endings to the therapeutic relationship: By not turning up for final appointments, becoming angry or blaming at the end of an intervention, or trying to prevent the ending by displaying dependency or recurrence of difficulties.

All these examples can pose difficulties but they do need to be dealt with in order to maintain the professional boundaries of your relationship. They can, in fact, be used to effect positive change for the client if dealt with in a therapeutic way. Indeed the process of working through issues as they arise in the relationship can be just as important an influence on the outcome of the therapy as the occupational intervention itself.

## Challenges of using the self in occupational therapy practice

It has been acknowledged by practising occupational therapists, that the use of self is vital to the outcomes of therapy and Taylor et al's (2009) research came to consider it to be the most important skill in occupational therapy practice. The same research also found that most participants did not feel they had sufficient training in this area of practice or that there was sufficient knowledge within occupational therapy practice. This was certainly my experience as a newly qualified practitioner and it took me many years of additional training and supervision in order to develop a skill set that I felt competent in utilising in practice. Despite this no one is perfect and gets it right all the time and some of the most valuable lessons I learnt were through some of the mistakes I made. The following examples illustrate what Taylor describes as 'empathic breaks' (Taylor 2008, p.123) in the relationship.

Empathic breaks can occur in the therapeutic relationship when 'a therapist fails to notice or understand a communication from a client or initiates a communication or behaviour that is perceived by the client as hurtful or insensitive' (Taylor 2008, p. 124). There are many reasons why this may happen. The examples I offer here relate to instances where the clients perceived that what I had said or how I had responded was not in the way they had wanted me to speak or respond.

The first example occurred when I first began working in a community mental health setting. A lady in her 30s was referred who was experiencing difficulties following the unexpected death of her husband a few months previously. This was the type of situation that as a young occupational therapist I found personally very challenging in respect of knowing how to 'be there' (Egan 1990, p. 57) with the client in distress and also worrying about saying the wrong thing or just not knowing how to respond to the client. On this occasion all my fears came home to roost! During the initial assessment, I felt overwhelmed by the emotional responses of the client and rather than allowing her to tell her story. I clearly said something that she perceived as me suggesting that she should be moving on in her grief. Not surprisingly, her response was less than positive and I immediately realised that I had in fact *said the wrong thing* and I needed to take responsibility for resolving or minimising this empathic break that had consequently occurred. I had no previous relationship with her to use in order to do this as this was the first time she had met me, so I felt that the only thing I could do at that stage was to apologise. Although this did not resolve the situation, she did agree to see me again the following week and during this time I used supervision to explore what had happened and how I could take this forward for the benefit of the client and our potential therapeutic relationship. The difficulties I had at that time in dealing with acute grief reactions were clearly my responsibility and reflected the stage in my life and lack of experience; it was an issue I was dealing with through supervision. In respect of the client and resolving the empathic break, I did go back and meet her; I acknowledged with her my part in what had happened and she was able to say that this was a common reaction she perceived from other people around her. We explored different options in terms of continuing her assessment and she decided she would prefer to be seen by someone older than herself that we were able to accommodate. Although this outcome did not allow for us to resolve the empathic break and continue to build up a positive therapeutic relationship, for her it was her preferred choice and I was able to reflect on what I had learned through this experience.

The second example revisits the issue of saying the wrong thing and demonstrates how as a more experienced and confident therapist I was able to use myself in the relationship more effectively in preventing and managing potential empathic breaks. In a day hospital setting, a young woman was referred who came to her initial appointment with her mother and sat hunched up in a corner, avoiding any eye contact, whilst her mother answered all the initial questions I asked. After a while she looked up at me in what seemed like a very direct/challenging way and said 'well, I just want you to know that if you say the wrong thing, I won't come back again!' I remember internally smiling at the irony of what she had obviously unknowingly said to me! However, by then I felt quite able to deal with this challenge. My response was to say that I was glad that she had been able to warn me but if we were to work together it was likely that I would say things that she did not like or saw as not agreeing with her, but the important thing for us would be that she told me when this happened and we could then talk about it. She clearly had not expected me to say this and just shrugged her shoulders. I did not expect her to come back the following week for her appointment that I had set with her mother, but she did, and she came on her own. This was the beginning of a very productive, albeit challenging, relationship where she would often test my boundaries and reactions through her comments and behaviours. Because of the relationship we developed I was able to use gentle, considered humour to challenge her very effectively and at the end of our intervention, where she was able to return to full-time work, she reflected herself on our first meeting, acknowledging how testing she had always been with me. On this occasion, the use of self was vital in engaging her in her desired occupation and consequently to the outcome of the therapy.

For me, developing effective skills in the use of self has not been an easy journey and I have had to learn a lot about myself along the way. In today's demanding health and social care environments where the complexity and challenges of clients' and carers' needs are ever growing I feel a re-focus on the use of self within an occupational milieu is needed in occupational therapy practices. This is necessary both for the outcomes of therapy and for the protection and self-care of occupational therapists who are often required to give so much of themselves through their work.

## Developing and supporting the use of self in occupational therapy practice

So how do occupational therapists develop and maintain these skills in practice? From my perspective it has been the result of a combination of further training and other continuing professional development (CPD) activities, effective and specific supervision in the use of self and learning from colleagues and clients.

Undertaking specific courses that incorporated the use of self-skills has been invaluable to my development, but I am not advocating that this is necessarily the appropriate route for everyone. I have realised over time that my preferred learning styles are of theorist and reflector (Honey and Mumford 1982), so a combination of undertaking CPD activities that have allowed me to learn the theory underpinning use of self and then reflecting (either on my own or with a supervisor) on how I use these within my occupationally focussed practice has worked well for me.

I have also learnt a lot from working with colleagues who I have thought exemplify the use of self in practice. These colleagues have come from a range of disciplines including psychology, nursing and social work as well as occupational therapy. I have also been very proactive at times throughout my career in seeking out supervision, specifically in respect to the use of self aspect of my practice. This has been particularly necessary when working with service users with complex needs such as eating disorders or personality disorders. Whatever your development needs are, in order to enhance the use of self in and maintain your occupational focus in practice, it is essential to develop a system of working which involves the use of reflection, self-awareness and appropriate supervision.

As practising occupational therapists in the United Kingdom, you will be aware of the requirements of the HPC for maintaining your registration and the need to work within your competency boundaries and within the areas of your professional domain. Furthering your self-awareness as a therapist and developing your skills in the use of self will only help to enhance your professional competency and effectiveness and enable you to act as a professional.

## Conclusion

This chapter has explored my personal perspective on how I have used a range of theories to support and develop the use of self within my own occupational therapy practice. The theory used has been drawn from psychotherapy and counselling theory that is a shared body of theory used by many professions. What is important in occupational therapy is how this use of self-theory is used with the overall aim of enhancing and impacting positively on the outcomes of occupationally focussed interventions. By remaining mindful of the occupational therapy theory umbrella presented in Chapter 3, it is possible for occupational therapists to see how the use of self can be used as the fabric that holds together a specific occupational therapy model and the approaches (shared with other professions) within contemporary practice. By implementing the use of self in this way, occupational therapists will then maintain their unique occupational focus in their practice.

## References

Bateman, A., Brown, D. and Pedder, J. (2000) *Introduction to Psychotherapy*, 3rd edn. London: Routledge.

Bion, W.R. (1961) *Experiences in Groups*. London: Tavistock Publications Limited.

Blair, S.E.E. and Daniel, M.A. (2006) An introduction to the psychodynamic frame of reference. In: *Foundations for Practice in Occupational Therapy*, ed. E.A.S. Duncan, 4th edn, pp. 233–253. Oxford: Elsevier.

College of Occupational Therapists (COT) (2010) *College of Occupational Therapists Code of Ethics and Professional Conduct*. London: College of Occupational Therapists.

Duncan, E.A.S. (2006) Skills and processes in occupational therapy. In: *Foundations for Practice in Occupational Therapy*, ed. E.A.S. Duncan, 4th edn, pp. 43–57. Oxford: Elsevier.

Egan, G. (1990) *The Skilled Helper*, 4th edn. California: Brooks/Cole Publishing Company.

Fidler, G.S. and Fidler, J.W. (1963) *Occupational Therapy: A Communication Process in Psychiatry*. New York: Macmillan.

Finlay, L. (1993) *Groupwork in Occupational Therapy*. Cheltenham Nelson Thornes Limited.

Finlay, L. (2004) *The Practice of Psychosocial Occupational Therapy*, 3rd edn. Cheltenham: Nelson Thornes Ltd.

Foulkes, S.H. (1983) *Introduction to Group-Analytic Psychotherapy: Studies in the Social Integration of Individuals and Groups*. London: Karnac Books.

Health Professions Council (HPC) (2008) Standards of conduct, performance and ethics. www.hpc-uk.org/publications (accessed March 2011).

Honey, P. and Mumford, A. (1982) *The Manual of Learning Styles*. Maidenhead: Peter Honey Publications.

Kielhofner, G. (2008) *Model of Human Occupation, Theory and Application*, 4th edn. Philadelphia: Lippincott, Williams and Wilkins.

Law, M., Baptiste, S. and Mills, J. (1995) Client centred practice: what does it mean and does it make a difference? *Canadian Journal of Occupational Therapy* 62(5), 250–257.

Mosey, A.C. (1981) *Occupational Therapy: Configuration of a Profession*. New York: Raven Press.

Mosey, A.C. (1986) *Psychosocial Components of Occupational Therapy*. New York: Raven Press.

Parker, D. (2006) The client-centred frame of reference. In: *Foundations for Practice in Occupational Therapy*, ed. E.A.S. Duncan, 4th edn, pp. 193–215. Oxford: Elsevier.

Rogers, R.C. (1951) *Client-Centered Therapy*. London: Constable.

Rogers, R.C. (1961) *On Becoming a Person*. London: Constable.

Taylor, R.R. (2008) *The Intentional Self: Occupational Therapy and Use of Self*. Philadelphia: F.A. Davis Company.

Taylor, R.R., Lee, S.W., Kielhofner, G. and Ketkar, M. (2009) Therapeutic use of self: A nationwide survey of practitioners' attitudes and experiences. *American Journal of Occupational Therapy* 63, 198–207.

Taylor, R.R. and Melton, J. (2009) Therapeutic use of self: a model of the intentional relationship. In: *Skills for Practice in Occupational Therapy*, ed. E.A.S. Duncan, pp. 123–144. Oxford: Elsevier.

Yalom, I. and Leszcz, M. (2005) *The Theory and Practice of Group Psychotherapy*, 5th edn. New York: Basic Books.

## Further reading

Taylor, R.R. (2008) *The Intentional Self: Occupational Therapy and Use of Self*. Philadelphia: F.A. Davis Company.

Taylor, R.R., Lee, S.W., Kielhofner, G. and Ketkar, M. (2009) Therapeutic use of self: a nationwide survey of practitioners' attitudes and experiences. *American Journal of Occupational Therapy* 63, 198–207.

# The Use of Theory in Practice: Some Practitioner Narratives

# Chapter 6

# Developing the use of the Model of Human Occupation in a mental health service

*Linda Keelan and Lisa John*

---

**Key points**

- Using an occupational therapy specific model enables occupationally focussed practice and clarifies professional reasoning
- A process of change requires sufficient time to embed theory into practice
- Commitment and support is required from managers to enable an effective change in practice
- Using an action research approach empowers staff to take ownership of a process of change

---

## Introduction

This chapter describes the journey towards more overt use of theory, still currently underway within an occupational therapy mental health service in Swansea, South Wales. The journey relates to developing the service's occupational therapy provision by underpinning it with the Model of Human Occupation (MOHO; Kielhofner 1985, 1995, 2002, 2008). This chapter is structured as follows:

- Setting the scene – a historical overview of the service
- The impetus for change:
  - Strategic
  - Operational
  - Practitioners
- Developing the use of theory in practice
- The journey to date and future plans

---

*Using Occupational Therapy Theory in Practice*, First Edition. Edited by Gail Boniface and Alison Seymour.
© 2012 Blackwell Publishing Ltd. Published 2012 by Blackwell Publishing Ltd.

It also intends to offer our interpretations (as the managers of the occupational therapy service) of our journey as a group of professionals attempting to embed our practice in the model, in order to enable an effective change in our practice.

## Setting the scene

The occupational therapists in Abertawe Bro Morgannwg University Health Board (ABMU) provide a range of community and hospital-based services for adults of working age and older adults. Prior to 2004, occupational therapy provision was provided as follows:

- Two adult community mental health teams (CMHTs) included two Senior 1 occupational therapists. Two further CMHTs had input from occupational therapists based in the hospital and day services.
- Within the hospital, there were five registered occupational therapists whose grades ranged from Basic Grade to Head III and four technical instructors. These covered three acute wards and three rehabilitation wards.
- Community services included a resource centre offering enhanced input for people whose needs could not be fully met through CMHT input alone. A Senior 1 occupational therapist and a technical instructor were based within the centre.

Within the hospital, there was also a heavy workshop area with 2.5 support grade occupational therapy staff. The workshop was accessed through the hospital-based occupational therapy staff in both adult and older people's services. Clients attending the workshop did so predominantly on a day basis from the community. Thus, the workshop was a community resource rather than a provision for in patients. This configuration of occupational therapy services was driven by organisational funding and service areas expectations; rather than current service need and priorities. Each of the registered staff took a care management role within the Care Programme Approach (CPA; Department of Health 1990) or key worker role and they were often seen to act generically. Thus, the clients these occupational therapists care managed represented a proportion of the team workload as opposed to being those with the highest level of occupational need. The in-patient staff worked with people during their time of admission, and there were issues of continuity of care. For example, a client discharged from the ward may have had an intervention that needed to be continued; however, the community-based occupational therapist may have had a different focus of role and different range of therapy skills. The in-patient occupational therapy staff experienced frustration in their roles, as there was a lack of follow-up, and high turnover of clients that left them feeling deskilled and undervalued. In addition, the expectations of the mental health service were rather traditional, with a perceived desire to limit occupational therapy to providing activities to relieve boredom on the ward, but not to be actively therapeutic. Thus, the service had not expanded to accommodate greater emphasis on community provision. Finally in addition to this rather traditional occupational therapy service provision, there were two areas where additional resources had been secured outside the mainstream funding of occupational therapy:

1. Firstly, within Her Majesty's Prison Swansea, a service was developed providing mental health services to the prison population experiencing mental distress, this included two occupational therapy staff – one clinical specialist and a technical instructor. These posts were funded separately through the Local Health Board, but were professionally part of the overall occupational therapy service.
2. Secondly, an occupational therapy service was also delivered within a local authority run rehabilitation facility, financed through Joint Flexibilities funding. This service consisted of a Senior 1 occupational therapist and four technical instructors. This team facilitated the rehabilitation and discharge of clients who had frequent re-admissions to the acute hospital wards. This team operated an in-reach process model, working closely with the ward team. Outcomes have been successful for this team and further funding has been ensured. From an occupational therapy perspective, this team evidenced the benefits of having a greater critical mass of occupational therapy staff that was not reflected anywhere else in the service. The make-up of the team was reviewed, resulting in an increase in the number of registered staff and a reduction in the number of support staff, to better meet the needs of the service users.

The older people's service, for adults over 65 with functional and organic disorders was similar but much smaller in staff numbers. It included three assessment wards, 4-day services and four continuing care wards. There were occupational therapy support staff working in isolation in day hospitals and the assessment ward, providing group-based interventions. Four occupational therapists ranging from Basic Grade to Senior 1 Grade focussed their input to the four older adult CMHTs. A clinical specialist working with complex cases worked across the whole patch and led the service. Each practitioner was professionally isolated, with little inter-relationship between support staff roles and the qualified occupational therapy roles. Referrals to the qualified occupational therapists were frequently triggered by service users' physical health issues, rather than mental health ones. The roles of the occupational therapists were frequently being defined by other professionals, rather than by occupational therapy. Referrals were also generated from specialist services, such as the Memory Clinic and Early Onset Dementia, where there were no dedicated occupational therapists, which led to inappropriate referrals.

Considering all this diversity of provision and expectations of the role of occupational therapy in the wider mental health service, we recognised that there were many challenges to delivering an occupational therapy service that was cohesive and consistent in its value base and practice, let alone one which was based in occupational therapy theory. This realisation resulted in a review of the whole occupational therapy service in mental health. The review demonstrated that our aims as occupational therapists were not being articulated in a way that was understood or seen as contributing to the attainment of our organisation's objectives. Thus, as the managers of the occupational therapy service we began by defining three key areas we felt could influence changes that were valued and visible to the wider organisation. These were as follows:

- To reduce the need for hospital admission
- To accelerate safe and early discharge from hospital
- To minimise disability and the impact of mental ill health

Other challenges that were highlighted in the review and of which we needed to be mindful were the lack of critical mass with a cohesive professional identity, difficulty in identifying levels of need as referral volume and nature varied widely according to other team members' perceptions of the role and contribution of occupational therapy to service users. The use of our professional skill mix was influenced largely by other professionals, so not always focussed on clients' occupational needs and did not reflect effective use of us as a scarce, unique professional resource. In terms of securing further resources, occupational therapy was not identified as a key player in service developments and where there was expansion, this often excluded occupational therapy. This was compounded by organisational arrangements, as occupational therapy was managed in a different directorate. The next three sections consider the need for our service to change and the potential impact of that change on various individual interests.

## The impetus for change: strategic

As the review of our occupational therapy service had demonstrated the nature of resourcing and developments within the service had resulted in patchy occupational therapy provision. In the adult service this meant that there were large CMHTs with individual, isolated occupational therapy practitioners, whilst other teams were without dedicated input. Evaluation of the input into these teams highlighted a lack of cohesion in provision and disparity in the role of the occupational therapists. This varied between team-based occupational therapy practitioners, whose roles were largely oriented around care management and generic team duties, and teams that utilised their sessional occupational therapists' input in high-volume work, such as anxiety management groups. Referral rates and throughput ranged hugely to reflect these disparities for us (the occupational therapy managers), which raised several questions:

- How were the occupational needs of clients being identified?
- As a scant resource, what was the impact of undertaking generic roles and interventions not specific to occupational therapy?
- How were referrers and service managers identifying the contribution of occupational therapy for the service and its users?

In addition, the in-patient settings had both a high patient turnover in the acute setting and a fairly static population of people with enduring mental health needs. How to focus and prioritise the allocation of staff resources to these very different client groups needed consideration. In examining this we were guided by where we could make the biggest difference, whilst also being aware of the *political* implications with our multi-disciplinary colleagues, hospital managers and occupational therapists who may have different views about us.

Occupational therapy services for older people were even more scant. Registered therapists of differing grades and experience were based in some, not all, community teams with others providing input to assessment units. Input into day hospitals and several wards were through support grade staff operating in isolation on a day-to-day basis. This raised issues of concern around clinical governance (see also Chapter 9 for a discussion on delegation and the role of occupational therapy support workers). The triggers for referral in this area were most frequently difficulties arising from co-existing physical health issues, or for the provision of activity. The challenge here was to develop and promote the contribution that occupational therapy could make to the service at earlier stages in diagnosis, and the value that addressing a range of occupational issues could have on the increased well-being of service users. From a value base, this service was very challenging. For example, occupational therapists discharged clients at the end of a treatment episode in order to keep caseloads at a number that allowed the therapists to work therapeutically and reflect active involvement. In contrast, some other multi-disciplinary colleagues held clients on an open caseload for the duration of their illness.

There were pressures to divert resources to give some input into newly developing areas and teams in both adult and older people's services. Usually there had been some additional posts in other staff groups, with requests for occupational therapy following, as gaps in service were identified. This challenge resulted in dissatisfaction on the part of team leaders and frustration for occupational therapists who were acutely aware that wherever they directed their input, a gap would form elsewhere.

Our colleagues and managers rarely understood our roles, as there was such variability and inconsistency. Where practitioners were carrying out similar generic roles, they were less challenged by multi-disciplinary colleagues or shared similar roles and duties. However, this did not support the case for actually having occupational therapy. In other areas, the occupational therapy role and practices had been defined by referrers, and referrers were doing so not on need but by interventions they knew we carried out. We were being judged and/or valued based on what we were *seen* to be capable of doing.

All of these factors led us to question and explore how effective our service was in meeting the occupational needs of our clients? And encouraged us to wonder, what would be the impact of not doing so? Within the local service a strong recovery focus was developing. The value and contribution of occupation within this was likely to be overlooked unless there was a clear identification and implementation of practices that could support this.

As a profession, our small research base that would be considered within evidence evaluated by National Institute of Clinical Excellence, and the resulting guidelines effectively meant that resources were directed locally in accordance with their recommendations. Without a clearly understood and recognised remit for occupational therapy, we were poorly placed to influence how guidelines are interpreted and put into practice.

The occupational therapy mental health service leads decided that there was a need to have a coherent service model and focus of delivery. We believed this would support us in defining our scope of service for occupational therapy, better defining and clarifying clinical roles and functions of occupational therapists and support staff, thus ensuring they identified and met the occupational needs of clients in all clinical service groupings. It was also a starting point for having the necessary dialogues with our managers and multi-disciplinary colleagues.

## The impetus for change: operational

As occupational therapy leads within this service we were passionate about occupational therapy, and having utilised the MOHO (Kielhofner 1985, 1995, 2002, 2008) within previous clinical practice, we felt that the model could provide a constructive framework when considering the future occupational therapy service focus.

At a similar time attendance by all senior staff at an Advanced Clinical Reasoning course contributed to the staff group considering where we are most effective. It caused us to question how we could deliver the greatest good to the largest amount of people, and made us revisit our duty of care. We felt it was important to link our professional changes and development into our organisation's three key areas (described in the preceding text) as a framework to define our unique input to others. Thus, our increased understanding of the service following the review all combined to direct some operational changes for us:

- Firstly, we relocated the majority of occupational therapy staff from both the clinical services to two bases; this relocation was supported by professional and service managers although it was acknowledged that this could have led to difficulties with multi-disciplinary and in fact occupational therapy staff.
- The occupational therapy referral form was then redesigned and structured using the MOHO (Kielhofner 1985, 1995, 2002, 2008). This then directed referrers to identify occupational issues, rather than defining problems or requesting particular interventions. These referrals were then sent to the two central occupational therapy bases, one for each clinical service. This process helped us with prioritisation of referrals based on occupational needs. It also enabled staff:case allocation by matching clinical complexity and the skills level of the occupational therapist, ensuring the most experienced therapists had the largest volume of complex cases. Additionally, it supported practitioners in developing and overtly demonstrating their clinical reasoning using the MOHO as a framework.

From a service perspective, provision began to be better focussed upon need, as opposed to the traditional location and availability of occupational therapists. Whilst some CMHTs were concerned that there may be less resource available, overall it ensured that the potential availability of occupational therapy intervention was more equitable across the whole service.

## The impetus for change: practitioners

The co-location of staff in shared bases afforded stronger links between the occupational therapists and support staff, who had previously been isolated in their practice. Opportunities for case discussion, sharing skills and problem-solving were enhanced. During this transition it seemed that the service apparently lacked a consistent value or philosophy base, which was then reflected in very different and diverse practices. Whilst practitioners were often highly valued multi-disciplinary team members as individuals, delivering occupational focussed interventions was not necessarily the priority of the team. Furthermore, there were vastly differing levels of familiarity, understanding and confidence with using any models of practice and applying occupational therapy theory into clinical work.

In order to help develop a shared value base within occupational therapy, links were developed with lecturing staff from a local university. A series of workshops were facilitated for the Band 7 occupational therapists focusing on updating knowledge of occupational therapy models and their use in practice. These workshops helped in opening a dialogue about existing practices and how they are framed, levels of comfort in using such models of practice within their clinical roles, and promoting practice that placed occupation at its core.

Clinical supervision sessions were also structured to support practitioners in developing their reasoning, alongside their new learning, and revisit profession-specific skills. At this stage, an exploration of occupational therapy models of practice indicated that further investigation into the MOHO (Kielhofner 1985, 1995, 2002, 2008) would be useful.

Some immediate issues became clear in regards to practitioners' confidence in using a professional model of occupational therapy to demonstrate and communicate their role. While some practitioners were able to use the associated standardised assessment tools, they were not confident in the theoretical understanding of the model to support the assessments' use in practice. There were also concerns about using other standardised assessments and frameworks such as the Claudia Allen assessment measure (Allen 1985) and how these may fit within the Human Occupation (Kielhofner 1985, 1995, 2002, 2008). Thus, from the practitioners' perspective, the introduction to the service of the MOHO was greeted as a potential help, but at the same time as a huge challenge and even a threat. Although as the managers of the occupational therapy service, we recognised the need to embed theory in practice, we also questioned our motivation for doing so and in particular in using this model. For example, were we leading from a position of dogmatic insistence that this model was right for us or were we leading from a position of recognising that this model could help us enable effective change in our practice?

With all of these questions, doubts and hope in mind, we nevertheless decided to go ahead and continue on our journey and try to embed occupational therapy theory into our practice via the MOHO.

## Developing the use of theory in practice

We recognised that in order to support practitioners in remaining focussed on working with clients in an occupational way, and not reverting to former habitual generic practices, further consolidation of knowledge and sharing of practice was required. Thus, in 2009 an action research project, which was instigated with the Band 7 occupational therapists, the two service managers and two occupational therapy lecturers began. One of the lecturers had previous experience of facilitating action research in occupational therapy services (Boniface et al 2008). The other had a wide experience within mental health services and had previously used the MOHO (Kielhofner 1985, 2002, 2008). This action research group formed the starting point of a more formal adoption of the model across the service.

Action research may be defined as research that is carried out with, rather than on the participants (Carr and Kemmis 1986; Reason 1994; Hart and Bond 1995; Heron 1996; Bray et al 2000; Meyer 2000). As well as action, this method of research includes cycles of reflection that the professional group felt was essential in the implementation of the model. Collaborative inquiry is a further form of action research and is 'essentially an emergent process' (Reason 1988, p. 19) and 'informative and explanatory' (Heron and Reason 2001, p. 183), as cited in Boniface et al (2008). The process is further described as a 'collaborative approach in the context that the researcher becomes a co-participant and participants become co-researchers' (Boniface et al 2008, p. 457). According to Meyer (2000), there are three elements central to action research:

- Its participatory nature.
- Its democratic nature.
- Its contribution to social science and social change, and it would be important to add to this list, its cyclical nature. Action research also offered the opportunity to develop a way of using theory to suit the needs of the staff group within the service.

Initial meetings were convened between the Band 7 practitioners and lecturers, acting as facilitators. It was decided that this grade of staff should be involved, as they were in positions to influence and bring about changes within the wider service and champion the use of the model within occupational therapy practice. The first task was to identify our aims. Initially, these were defined as follows:

1. Investigate the potential for change in occupational therapy practice to establish the occupational focus of practice via the use of the Model of Human Occupation.
2. Identify the potential links between the use of the model and other theories in use within the service at the time.
3. Embed client-centred theory in the practice of the therapists.

Whilst establishing these aims, a research bid was submitted to try to secure funding to support the project. Unfortunately, this was unsuccessful; however, the group decided with the support of the service managers and the university staff to continue with the project regardless of external funding.

The action research took the format of a focussed group experience, sharing practice issues, concerns relating to the introduction of the model and its impact upon workloads. With consent from the occupational therapists these sessions were audio-recorded and transcribed by the facilitators, who sent these out to the group between sessions. The facilitators analysed the transcripts, identified emerging themes that were related to the research aims and sent these to the group for consideration. The emerging themes and actions were interwoven.

An initial common theme was the use of the model's language and comfort with articulating the model. The first action was for each practitioner to identify and present a case to their peer group using the model's terminology. This process highlighted practitioners' level of anxiety and confidence in applying the model to a case study. To address this, smaller peer groups were formed fulfilling the same function and a monthly consultation session was made available for all the practitioners desiring individual case discussion. This improved morale and gave permission for practitioners to be open and honest about their level of developing knowledge and areas for further investigation. The effect this had was to make the research group experience more positive.

Organisational and personal barriers to implementing the model continued to be an emerging theme throughout the process. The perceived value of the model and how it could be of benefit to the client, and the perception of a better service provision by our multi-disciplinary colleagues was questioned. At the same time, there were areas of opportunity and service expansion. This provided a means of establishing practice and service provision that was defined and delivered using an occupationally focussed model. In these areas, the contribution of occupational therapists working both occupationally and in an outcome focussed way was visibly different from other professionals' input, and the outcomes began to be recognised at a clinical and management level. For example, people with long-term and enduring mental health needs were successfully returned from high cost specialist placements, undergoing rehabilitation within the local hospital and were then being placed in non-health settings within the community. This helped to promote a better understanding across the service of our key functions and the contribution that our input could make, and resulted in some further increases in occupational therapy staffing resource.

A further barrier was staff feeling that they needed permission to take time away from face to face clinical duties in order to become more familiar with the model. This issue was addressed by the allocation of time for continuous professional development. Relevant literature and up-to-date assessment tools were purchased and made available across the service bases. The support of the service managers in giving permission and the opportunity to allow these developments was crucial to the success of the emerging integration of theory into practice.

During the initial action research meetings, another common theme identified was the practitioners' lack of integration of theoretical knowledge into clinical practice. It became evident that this involved more than just being able to administer a MOHO-based assessment tool. Recognising this gap in theoretical knowledge, it was decided that peer-led book groups would be developed (similar to journal club formats) to enable the reading and discussion of specific chapters from the latest MOHO publication (Kielhofner 2008). This process continues to date, and is also incorporated into the supervision process. For example, one occupational therapist prepared an in-depth case analysis that presented the client's strengths and needs in a structured occupational framework that reflected the practitioner's growing level of knowledge, understanding and synthesis of the model into practice. This format has since been adopted by her peers. The book groups are now being rolled out to the Bands 5 and 6 occupational therapists and are facilitated by the Band 7 occupational therapists who are now beginning to feel confident in their understanding and use of theory underpinning the model.

It has been apparent that the developing use of the model is of its nature cyclical, with a close inter-relationship among knowledge, practice and supervision. This has taken, to date, a period of 2 years to allow people to adjust and truly change their practice at a pace that was sustainable for the service, and acknowledged individuals' capacity for change. This process remains ongoing.

## The journey to date and the future

The experience of engaging with the model has enabled a significant change in practice for both individual occupational therapists and the occupational therapy service. In the management of caseloads, a greater occupational focus, supported by the supervision and caseload management process, has resulted in being more outcome focussed and a greater throughput for clients and for the service. As a consequence, clients receiving occupationally focussed interventions are involved in the service specifically for these needs and are more equipped to live their lives, as opposed to being held within a service because they have a condition. This is reflected within the CPA, where the occupational therapists support this process by targeting their assessment and interventions specifically in areas of occupational need.

The Band 7 occupational therapists involved in this journey represented the most senior clinicians within the service. As we were seeking to shape the whole of occupational therapy provision, clearly we now need to involve the whole staff group in this change in practice and this is the basis of the next cycle of action and includes the following:

- Awareness workshops for all staff to raise understanding of the model, the rationale for its use within the service, and exploration of what is now required to roll this process out.
- Development of book groups for Bands 5 and 6 occupational therapists to begin the process of integrating theory into practice.
- Incorporating the use of the model more overtly within the cascading supervision structures between the grades of occupational therapy staff.

- Raising awareness of this process and the use of the model to support staff and deciding the delineation of use of the theory within their role. (We are aware occupational therapists in Gloucestershire have already considered this issue – see Chapter 9.)
- Adoption of a priority screening tool for referrals to the occupational therapy service based on the model.
- Development of organisational initial assessment based on the theory of the model.
- Development of a training package that can be utilised by existing and new staff.
- Incorporation of the model into service user information.

## Conclusion

This chapter has described a process of change. The process is aimed at developing the use of theory through using an occupational therapy model of practice to underpin occupational therapy in an area that was becoming increasingly under pressure to deliver generic mental health interventions within multi-disciplinary services. It has outlined some of the challenges we faced both from a service and individual practitioner perspective and describes how the process of engaging in an action research project has empowered the staff to take ownership of this process of change. What we now have is a more targeted occupational therapy service, which contributes to the more generic mental health interventions in an occupationally focussed or based way.

The increased confidence in using theory in practice and the greater focus on occupational-based interventions has had a huge impact on the occupational therapy team. Many have reported greater job satisfaction and clarity of role within their multi-disciplinary teams. They have expressed a stronger ability to articulate their clinical reasoning in both multi-disciplinary and multi-agency settings, and are better able to evidence when clients have needs that require occupational therapy, or conversely when occupational therapy is not required. This has been further evidenced through feedback from other team members about the experience that clients have had whilst engaged with an occupational therapist. Staff have also reported feeling validated when hearing their multi-professional colleagues discussing clients using their professional language around occupations in context.

Several new posts have been recently resourced for occupational therapists in areas where there had not been any tradition of occupational therapy involvement. We believe that these developments have been possible due to the following:

- Greater confidence in defining the outcomes of occupational therapy
- Quality issues relating to the client experience
- Having a coherent and consistent model of service regardless of clinical or geographical area
- Confidence in conveying this to planners and budget holders who understood and evaluated our input differently

We recognise that there has been significant growth and change within the service, and are proud of the journey that the occupational therapists have taken, with its highs and lows and capacity to stick with it when going back to comfortable and familiar practice would have been so easy. As a journey, we will continue to strive to provide the best possible service for our clients, and support the development of services that consider and attend to the occupational daily lives of clients within our community.

## Acknowledgements

Thanks are due to Gail Boniface and Alison Seymour for their engagement with the team in the participatory action research process.

## References

Allen, C.K. (1985) *Occupational Therapy for Psychiatric Diseases: Measurement and Management of Cognitive Disabilities*. Boston: Little, Brown, and Company.

Boniface, G., Fedden, T., Hurst, H., Mason, M., Phelps, C., Reagon, C. and Waygood, S. (2008) Using theory to underpin an integrated occupational therapy service through the Canadian Model of Occupational Performance. *British Journal of Occupational Therapy*, 71(12), 531–539.

Bray, J.N., Lee, J., Smith, L.L. and Yorks, L. (2000) *Collaborative Inquiry in Practice*. Thousand Oaks, CA: Sage.

Carr, W. and Kemmis, S. (1986) *Becoming Critical: Knowing through Action Research*. Victoria: Deakin University.

Department of Health (1990) *The Care Programme Approach for People with Mental Illness, Referred to Specialist Psychiatric Services*. London: Department of Health.

Hart, E. and Bond, M. (1995) *Action Research for Health and Social Care: A Guide to Practice*. Buckingham: Open University Press.

Heron, J. (1996) *Cooperative Inquiry: Research into the Human Condition*. London: Sage.

Heron, J. and Reason, P. (2001) The practice of cooperative inquiry: research 'with' rather than 'on' people. In: *Handbook of Action Research*, eds P. Reason and H. Bradbury, pp. 179–188. London: Sage.

Kielhofner, G. (1985) *A Model of Human Occupation: Theory and Application*. Baltimore: Lippincott, Williams and Wilkins.

Kielhofner, G. (1995) *A Model of Human Occupation*, 2nd edn. Baltimore: Lippincott, Williams and Wilkins.

Kielhofner, G. (2002) *A Model of Human Occupation*, 3rd edn. Baltimore: Lippincott, Williams and Wilkins.

Kielhofner G. (2008) *A Model of Human Occupation: Theory and Application*, 4th edn. Baltimore: Lippincott, Williams and Wilkins.

Meyer, J. (2000) Using qualitative methods in health related action research. *British Medical Journal* 320(7228), 178–181.

Reason, P. (ed.) (1988) *Human Inquiry in Action*. London: Sage.

Reason, P. (ed.) (1994) *Participation in Human Inquiry*. London: Sage.

# Further reading

Boniface, G., Fedden, T., Hurst, H., Mason, M., Phelps, C., Reagon, C. and Waygood, S. (2008) Using theory to underpin an integrated occupational therapy service through the Canadian Model of Occupational Performance. *British Journal of Occupational Therapy*, 71(12), 531–539.

# Chapter 7

# Using Reed and Sanderson's Model of Adaptation through Occupation: a journey

*Karen Lewis and Sharon James*

---

**Key points**

- Implementing an occupational therapy professional model represents a journey into clarity of occupational thinking
- Occupational therapy outcome measures should measure changes in occupational performance
- Occupational performance-based outcome measures can be used to clinically reason the involvement of the service user in specific occupational interventions

---

## Introduction

This chapter describes the journey of the occupational therapy service within Morriston Hospital, Swansea, into the implementation of an occupational therapy professional model and the consequential development of an associated outcome measure. It is written by two authors who still work in the hospital, and they describe their separate but linked journeys in the use of occupational therapy theory. The chapter also outlines the process of the model's implementation and describes how the service developed a stronger sense of professional identity and a clearer structure for documentation.

The journey began when occupational therapy professional models (Reed 1984) heralded a new era for occupational therapy practice particularly for myself, the first author. For me occupation had suddenly become a talking point, a valid vehicle for delivering health care. Occupation became *respectable* with its own philosophical base and concepts. When I first encountered it, I saw Adaption through Occupation (Reed and Sanderson 1983) as something that could enable occupational therapists to structure and explain the use of occupation in their practice. Later, Reed (1984) clarified this for me. At the core of the model was the use of occupation, and its key role in enabling people to develop, restore or engage in their everyday activities. Reed (1984) discusses the nature of change and the need for the profession to address change and

---

*Using Occupational Therapy Theory in Practice*, First Edition. Edited by Gail Boniface and Alison Seymour.
© 2012 Blackwell Publishing Ltd. Published 2012 by Blackwell Publishing Ltd.

re-examine its values and philosophical base. The theme of change was also evident in her view that a model should guide action and reflect changes in the environment in which it is used. The 1992 and 1999 versions of *Concepts of Occupational Therapy* (Reed and Sanderson) gave us more food for thought when it was proposed that occupational therapists should select a model that will guide practice that most closely fits our ideals and values as a profession.

Although the Model of Adaptation through Occupation may not be perfect, it does have much to offer the practising occupational therapist. In order to understand what this might entail, it is useful for us to familiarise ourselves with the basic assumptions and concepts. Reed and Sanderson (1999, p. 226) suggest that the best way to gain an understanding is to examine the basic assumptions and the 'three major concepts' of the model. With this in mind I (first author) will attempt to articulate my understanding of the basic assumptions of the Model of Adaptation Through Occupation in the next section.

## Model of Adaptation through Occupation: basic assumptions and concepts

From the birth of this concept to the current time, occupation continues to be the quintessence of Adaptation through Occupation. Within the model, the definition of occupation has evolved over the years. In the early years, occupations were thought of as structured and definitive. Although descriptions such as 'goal-directed' (Reed 1984, p. 497) activities that engage a person's time and attention and 'meaningful and purposeful' (Reed 1984, p. 498) led us to view occupations in a prescriptive way, we were at least talking about occupations. However taken in the context of an occupational therapy practitioner working in an environment where the medical approach was viewed as the only valid practice in patient care, the term *occupation* and the assumption that occupation was central to all existence, was almost heretical to the medical establishment and subsequently quite revolutionary. Even at its inception, Adaptation through Occupation inspired occupational therapists who were struggling to fit a holistic and person-centred approach into their care. Later definitions of occupations were far less prescriptive. Occupations had evolved to be 'naturally occurring events . . . because they support life and . . . promote adaptation to the environment . . . facilitating growth and development through learning and mastery' (Reed and Sanderson 1999, p. 33). This view broadens the definition and meaning of occupations and thus the model began to become a *model for* rather than a *model of* (see Chapter 2) our profession for us. No longer are occupations associated with defined activities, they are now life events that live and surround us from birth to death. They support us in enabling us to fulfil our needs in the environment that we choose/adapt to be our own.

Whether you view occupations as life events or meaningful activities, Adaptation through Occupation divides occupations into the sub-categories of self-maintenance, productivity and leisure, as outlined in Chapter 3. However, the focus of choice lies with the individual. Self-maintenance, productivity and leisure have fluidity and can interchange by the moment. An occupation may be perceived as productive by one individual, and leisure by another. In addition, an individual may change their perceptions of occupations, activities and tasks undertaken, often driven by influences around and within them.

The inter-relationship of self-maintenance, productivity and leisure is also influenced by the need of the individual to have a balance of occupations to facilitate health and well-being. Balance of occupations is viewed as another core assumption in the Model of Adaptation through Occupation. To understand the term *balance*, it is essential to accept that this does not mean an equal balance in self-maintenance, productivity and leisure. Balance in occupations is defined by Reed and Sanderson (1999, p. 34) as spending 'some time in all activities on a regularly recurring basis'. Some people may flourish by engaging in occupations that focus on self-maintenance and leisure pursuits, productivity playing a minor part in their lives. Others would feel unhappy with this *balance* and would prefer larger amounts of productivity and less self-maintenance and leisure. As a practitioner (first author), when trying to implement this model, I struggled with trying to identify whether there was a balance of occupations in my patients' lives. How could I gain this information during assessment without influencing or confusing my patients? I eventually found that asking open questions such as 'how do you spend your day' would enable the patients to describe their occupations in their own words. Of course patients did, at times, give me an hourly description of their activities! However, on the whole they would talk generally about their daily lives. Following this, I would ask them 'which of your activities would you think of as a job or role as opposed to those that you do just for enjoyment'. That did help to identify productivity and leisure, self-maintenance being easier to identify from the outset. Over the years, I realised that an imbalance of occupations was far easier to recognise. During the assessment process I regularly asked patients 'how do you feel in yourself'? Those who reflected feelings of unhappiness, being devalued or having a loss of self-confidence would, when asked about how they spent their day throw the question back at me or answer negatively in terms of 'can't do anything as I am' and often became emotional and tearful. Here was an example of the close link between well-being and occupational balance. This is where as an occupational therapist, I could use my skills and influence well-being.

The model's next assumption is concerning the environment and the process of adaptation. Reed and Sanderson (1983, 1999) believe that adaptation is a concept central to occupational therapy. Adaptation through Occupation articulates the concept of adaptation and supports the belief that a person can adapt themselves to shape their future through the use of occupations. An individual has the capacity to adapt or alter themselves and/or the environment in which he or she carries out occupations in order to achieve health, well-being and fulfilment. The final concept of my list of three is that all occupations are determined by the environment. Occupations, and our ways of carrying them out, are developed and exist due to the environment in which we live. Occupations not supported by the environment are phased out, for example, writing letters as a means of communicating information to friends/family is being replaced by mobile phones, texting and electronic communication. However, environments can also assist occupation (Reed and Sanderson 1983, 1999). For example, individuals unable to perform writing tasks due to performance skill deficits can be enabled to communicate through electronic methods of communication.

In the early version of the model, Reed (1984) discussed five performance skills required to carry out occupations. Later publications merged these categories into three: sensory/motor, cognitive and psychosocial. This did simplify the use of the model in practice as assessments could thus be divided up into three sections (environment, performance skills and occupations); each of which could be sub-divided into three further sections as follows:

- *Environment*: physical, psycho-biological and sociocultural
- *Performance skills*: motor/sensory, cognitive and intra- inter-personal skills
- *Occupations*: self-maintenance, productivity and leisure

This pragmatic revision did much to guide action and adapt to clinicians' need to develop their own assessments based on the model to facilitate application of the use of theory whilst using the problem-solving process.

## The development of the Model of Adaptation through Occupation within an occupational therapy service

Having begun to get to grips with the theory of the model in 1991, the Occupational Therapy service within Morriston Hospital in Swansea embarked on a journey during which there was no turning back. This was the year that myself (first author) and two colleagues decided to find out what 'the fuss was all about' in respect of occupational therapy professional models. We had been questioned frequently by students as to 'which model we used' and if we admitted to not utilising a 'model' then 'why not' nagged the students.

Around this time, the local occupational therapy lecturers were organising a workshop for practitioners who needed to understand the way in which occupational therapy professional models could guide practice. Before we knew it, the three of us had been volunteered to attend the workshop and feedback to the Head of Department.

We all expected to find the workshop unenlightening and confirm our notions that these models were yet another 'new' idea doomed for failure that would not apply to us, working in an acute setting. How wrong we were!

The workshop, held over 3 days, introduced us to a way of working that we thought had been buried in the desire to earn credibility in the medical world by providing regimented treatment activity for patients and supplying items of equipment for patients to define our role within 'the firm'. Occupational therapy professional models now seemed to have a purpose; they could create and guide and articulate a unique identity for occupational therapists. As a result of much debate and questioning, we were drawn to the Model of Adaptation through Occupation (Reed and Sanderson 1983, 1999). We felt that the problem-solving approach inherent in this model would reflect the approach used by the occupational therapists in our acute setting and would be comfortable to adopt in our environment. We all felt that here was an inspirational concept that would explain and guide our practice as occupational therapists. No longer would we cringe when asked 'what work do you do', we would have a definitive explanation that would set us aside from our physiotherapy colleagues.

The next step was to provide feedback to our Head of Department. Thanks to her vision, she agreed to support our ideas to develop the occupational therapy service in Morriston. A steering group was formed and the next stage was agreed, that is, to decide upon which occupational therapy professional model to use to guide us in the development of our service.

## Implementation of the model

We started by researching relevant literature, attending more workshops and bench-marking other services. The local university occupational therapy staff were extremely supportive providing advice, information and contributing to discussions. Finally, we presented the findings to our senior staff and agreed that the Model of Adaptation through Occupation would support the occupational therapy service and contained the *tools* that would enable us to structure and develop our service.

The next stage was to market the concept of Adaptation through Occupation to the staff group as a whole and decide upon its use in practice. It was decided to arrange a study day where staff could debate and consider the proposal.

## The debate

### June 1992

The study day was led by a colleague and myself (the first author). Two tutors from the local occupational therapy course also attended as facilitators. Discussions took place around models, specifically around their use and meaning. There was much debate about the nature of the occupational therapy service in Morriston. The staff felt it important that any change should bring benefits to the service in terms of quality to patient interventions. They were anxious about this new concept, the jargon and perceived additional paperwork. Following vigorous debate, it was agreed that an occupational therapy professional model *could* have something to offer the service. The staff were keen to develop a service that would reflect their working practice and which was meaningful to them as occupational therapists. The consensus of staff was that the Model of Adaptation through Occupation lent itself to our acute setting. The model's concepts were meaningful and the language easily understood. The problem-solving process was also inherent in the model, already an integral aspect to the working practice of the occupational therapists. As a result, it was decided to adopt the Model of Adaptation through Occupation as a pilot study for 6 months, following which there would be an opportunity for a review.

The discussions had highlighted a *gap* in our use of the problem-solving process in Morriston. Feedback from students and new staff had questioned the lack of a structured initial assessment. All occupational therapy staff reported that they carried out an initial interview/assessment. However, each practitioner seemed to follow their own format that not only made it very confusing for the student occupational therapists or newly qualified staff but also did not document any active engagement of the patient in the assessment process. It was agreed to structure an initial assessment form guided by the Model of Adaptation through Occupation that would describe a patient's occupations, identify, skills and competencies, and through dialogue with the patient highlight occupational areas of concern for the patient. This would enable the occupational therapist to plan and direct patient-centred intervention. More detailed information and study followed into the Model of Adaptation through Occupation, and in August 1992, an occupational therapy initial assessment form and intervention form were born out of the model.

Looking back, once an initial start had been made using the model of practice seemed to take on a life of its own. The 6-months pilot came and went, and staff were actively engaging in implementing actions guided by Adaptation through Occupation and seemed to forget that an evaluation was needed!

## *A reflective digression*

I (first author) took the opportunity whilst writing this chapter to return to the staff who were part of this process to gather their recollections of this time in their career.

I was quite surprised to discover that only three members of staff remained working within Morriston that were at the inception of our new ways of working. The three staff members were happy to share their memories, reflecting back to 1992. From our discussions, themes emerged around their thoughts, feelings and professional opinions.

The initial thoughts they articulated were around the credibility of having a defined role and purpose to interventions. One member of staff who was a very junior occupational therapist at the time remembered how this service development indicated that Morriston was a forward moving service. All three remembered feeling slightly daunted by the prospect of change and moving forward. Feelings around more documentation, more work and changes to a well-established system contributed to their anxieties. However, on a more positive note, it was felt that the implementation starting with the study day was successful and enabled staff to articulate their concerns within a supportive environment.

Reflecting on the Model of Adaptation through Occupation, all three agreed that the nature of this occupational therapy professional model was particularly meaningful within their clinical settings. Two of the staff were familiar with the Model of Human Occupation, Kielhofner (1985) and recalled leaving the study day thankful that we were not proposing to be guided by this model, which they perceived as less adaptable to the fast pace of an acute setting. Comparing current practice with historical practice, the staff felt that there was now more structure, which is helpful to junior staff and gives clarity to the problem-solving process. The development of the initial assessment form was something they welcomed as it is now such an integral part of practice, they could not envisage being without it! They all felt that following the implementation of new ways of working, occupations and the balance of occupations had come alive as concepts. Although there were acknowledgements that within the acute setting, clinical areas did not have the resources in terms of staff time to address imbalance issues effectively, it was agreed that it is the role of the occupational therapist to identify imbalance in a patient's occupations so that strategies can be implemented or at least highlighted. In using the model, the occupational therapist has the opportunity during a patient's admission to highlight an imbalance of occupations and introduce this concept to patients, planting seeds of thought for patients to consider and thus to empower them to adapt their occupations and participate in interventions during rehabilitation whilst as an in-patient or following discharge home.

These recollections provide us with the benefit of hindsight and reassure us that the unmapped road of service development has indeed led us to greener pastures!

Following this diversion into the future, I (first author) take us back to 1994 when it was time to evaluate the implementation of our model.

## February 1994

A formal evaluation of the Model of Adaptation through Occupation was undertaken. Questionnaires were sent to all the Occupational Therapy staff to elicit their opinions on their understanding of 'the model', the appropriateness to the work setting, the re-modelled assessment and intervention forms, their usefulness and applicability.

## The debate outcome

There was an extremely positive response to the Model of Adaptation through Occupation. Staff felt that it helped to structure their assessments and interventions and gave them a sense of identity. The content of the assessment forms was supported; however, the format was identified as requiring further work. The intervention forms we had devised were unpopular and the staff felt that work was being duplicated. Further work had to be done here! The staff also requested induction for all new occupational therapy staff into the model and our service development.

## A further amendment to the assessment form July 1995

Further work by the authors had resulted in an amended assessment form. The evaluation in 1994 had highlighted the diversity of clinical areas within Morriston at that time. Specialist areas such as neuro-rehabilitation and palliative medicine had very different requirements of their assessment tools. Neuro-rehabilitation wanted a large section to record performance skills whilst palliative medicine requested a large section to record the organic environment. Each of these clinical areas was engaged in their commitment to be guided by the model and its concepts; however, the overall format needed to be amended to adapt to the needs of the individual clinical areas. We engage in client-centred approach in respect of our patients/service users. However, we perhaps forget that services that have similar needs and uniformity, whether via documentation or practice, can conflict with the individualised nature of service provision.

Thus, the intervention form underwent a complete revamp. It underwent a metamorphosis to become an intervention/outcome form. The journey into this transformation is detailed in the next part of this chapter by the second author Sharon James. She will describe the processes that led to the adoption of an outcome measure, embedded in the Model of Adaptation through Occupation.

## The Morriston Occupational Therapy Outcome Measure

### Why was MOTOM developed?

The honest answer to why Morriston Occupational Therapy Outcome Measure (MOTOM) was initially developed was that I (second author) was undertaking a diploma in supervisory management in 1993 that required the participants to undertake a project. I wanted to utilise the opportunity to undertake a piece of work that would be of practical benefit to the department, rather than just an academic exercise. Thus, following a discussion with my manager, it was agreed that the most beneficial project would be to evaluate outcome measures in order to identify the one that would be suitable to use within the service.

The project aimed to review the range of existing outcome measures, then present the findings to the occupational therapy staff and information department in order to identify the preferred method of measuring outcome for the occupational therapy service. Key issues for consideration were the range of clinical specialities within Morriston and the supporting community hospitals, and the need for any outcome measure to be congruent with the philosophy and documentation used within the service that had been recently developed around the Model of Adaptation through Occupation (Reed and Sanderson 1992). The agreed criteria for an outcome measure were as follows:

- It was quick to administer.
- It was simple and not open to misinterpretation.
- It should give relevant and accurate information.
- It should incorporate the views of the patient.
- It should measure all issues addressed by the occupational therapists.
- It should be appropriate for use in all clinical areas.

I reviewed existing outcome measures utilising literature, occupational therapy education and experiences of occupational therapy managers within the South Wales locality in an attempt to find the perfect outcome measure that met the above criteria. Whilst all acknowledged the growing importance of outcome measures, very few were being used in practice, and the range of outcome measures was limited to performance skill indices such as the Barthel Index (Mahoney and Barthel 1965), patient satisfaction surveys or goal attainment scaling. Activities of daily living (ADL) indices such as the Barthel, whilst being widely recognised and considered by many to be the gold standard, were not considered appropriate for our purpose of measuring the outcome of our concentration on occupations, or for use in acute settings due to the need to assess a patient then reassess at a later date. Perhaps more importantly though, as a staff group we were recognising the restrictive nature of ADL indices and began to feel constrained by the limitations of measuring only those items that appear on a predetermined list (Eakin 1991; MacAvoy 1991; Unsworth 1993). This limited approach to what was measured did not fit with the philosophy of occupational therapy being client centred, occupationally focused and addressing those issues that are important to the individual service user, and the holistic nature of assessment as framed by the Model of Adaptation through Occupation (Reed and Sanderson 1992). Supporting this, occupational therapists' use of outcome indices such as the Barthel Index is often at the request of other professionals, and that whilst the benefits of using such a well-recognised tool can be obvious, it is important for our profession to use a tool that measures the full extent of the benefit of occupational therapy itself, not merely performance skills.

It was whilst visiting a research therapist in Coventry that I was made aware of the newly (at the time) developed Canadian Occupational Performance Measure (COPM) (Law et al 1994). I was extremely excited by this discovery, as it seemed at last there was an outcome measure that was meaningful and really measured what was important to occupational therapists. I could also see that a measure of outcome could be linked to an occupational therapy professional model, and this inspired me further to think about developing an outcome measure that could be linked to the Model of Adaptation through Occupation (Reed and Sanderson 1983, 1992, 1999) that we were using, in the same way that COPM (Law et al 1994) had been developed from The Canadian Model of Occupational Performance (Townsend et al 1997). Not only would this make the measure easier to integrate into the existing documentation but also it would, more importantly, make it congruent with the theories that now guided and structured our practice. Consultation with colleagues confirmed that the approach and philosophy of COPM was desirable, but due to the very acute nature of many of the clinical teams, the process needed to be less time consuming. In addition to the process being simplified, the service required a single outcome for each patient seen in order to utilise the outcomes in service evaluation. It became evident that an outcome measure would need to be designed and developed, inspired by COPM and how that tool had been developed as a development of The Canadian Model of Occupational Performance (Townsend et al 1997), but to be integrated with the Model of Adaptation through Occupation (Reed and Sanderson 1992) for our purposes.

Therefore, I decided that an outcome measure would be developed utilising the principles of COPM, but adapted to meet the criteria outlined earlier, making it suitable for use in a fast paced, acute service. It was agreed that the measure would comprise a rating of ability before and after occupational therapy intervention. The method of identification of areas of performance to measure, the use of an importance weighting, the rating scale used, the service user contribution to the process and the method of documentation were all areas that required further development in our setting.

## What to measure

The initial stage of COPM (Law et al 1994) whereby the service users identify the difficulties they are experiencing within specific occupational performance areas was in part mirrored by the model-based initial assessment used in our service. The development of the more structured assessment based on the Model of Adaptation through Occupation (Reed and Sanderson 1983, 1992, 1999) ensured the holistic assessment of all areas of occupational performance, thereby identifying what was important to an individual service user. The structure of the assessment facilitated the identification under the categories of self-care, productivity and leisure, as in COPM. The joint identification of problems by the therapist and service user was felt to be more appropriate in the range of clinical areas in the service due to the acute nature of many of these areas. The client-led structure of COPM has been found to be most effective where there is time to develop the client–therapist relationship (Waters 1995), and where service users have sufficient insight and cognitive ability (Toomey et al 1995; Ward et al 1996). Ward et al (1996) also noted a reluctance of service users to voice concerns regarding their abilities for fear of a delayed discharge in settings such as ours. Therefore, it was agreed that the areas to be rated would be jointly agreed by the therapist and the service user based on the outcome of the initial and subsequent assessments.

## Development of MOTOM took a long time

The development of MOTOM took place over several years. The initial stage comprised the development of a pilot tool in collaboration with senior colleagues in the service in June 1994. This version of MOTOM used a 4-point rating scale to rate ability before and after intervention. Problems identified were initially under the categories of environment, occupations and performance. Details of problems and outcomes were documented on an outcome form. An outcome score for each problem was calculated as the difference in the pre- and post-intervention scores, and a single outcome score was calculated as the mean of the individual scores. Where there were no relevant issues for occupational therapy, there was a code to denote this. The tool was piloted for a period of 3 months and then evaluated. The evaluation comprised a survey via questionnaire completed by all the occupational therapists using the tool. The findings of the survey were evaluated, and following collaboration with a clinical research scientist and a medical sociologist, version 2 of MOTOM, was developed. The amendments included the following:

- The use of an outcome calculation form.
- The introduction of a 10-point importance weighing scale.
- Change in the rating scale to allow calculation with an importance weighing, that is, a scale of 1–4 rather than 0–3.
- Detailed explanation of the scoring system.
- Additional codes where occupational therapy intervention was not appropriate.

It was upon the advice of the academics consulted that the importance weighting, similar to that used in COPM, was introduced to MOTOM.

The amended tool, version 2, was implemented in March 1995 and piloted for a further 3 months. The evaluation of this version was undertaken via focus groups with each clinical team to allow more detailed discussions and in-depth evaluation. This led to further amendments, with version 3 of MOTOM having the following changes:

- Combination of the intervention form and the outcome calculation form to reduce duplication of documentation.
- The introduction of further outcome codes to accurately reflect why occupational therapy intervention was not appropriate for some service users.
- The amendment of the importance weighting to a 3 point rather than a 10-point scale that could be allocated following general discussion with service users rather than them having to select the specific rating.

Version 3 of MOTOM was then implemented and used for several months. A sample of documentation from each clinical team including the initial assessment form and the intervention/outcome form was audited. The findings of the audit resulted in further amendments to the intervention/outcome form with improved guidance for the therapists using the tool. These included the need to document problems in terms of the occupational performance ability or level of functional deficit rather than just state that there was a problem in a particular area. Similarly the need to document outcomes in terms of how the service user was now able to function rather than just a statement of what intervention had been completed. This point in the development of MOTOM marked the recognition of a significant shift in thinking that was required by the therapists. The difficulty in changing working practices that had become ingrained in practice proved more difficult than subsequent teachings to newly qualified therapists. As occupational therapy education has promoted the use of occupational therapy professional models, the understanding of the philosophy of occupational therapy and the key role of occupations as central to our practice have come to underpin that practice. However, many practitioners had undertaken their occupational therapy courses before this time and whilst they were experts in the technical delivery of occupational therapy assessment and intervention, struggled with the shift in thinking that allows explanation of what we do in occupational terms. I (second author) was certainly one of the latter types of therapist, yet through the involvement in implementing the model and developing the outcome measure have come to value the benefit of that underpinning philosophy.

Following the continued use of MOTOM in the service, a study day that aimed to share the experience of implementing the Model of Adaptation through Occupation (Reed and Sanderson 1992) and MOTOM as a method of measuring outcome was held in 1996. The study day prompted interest in MOTOM that led to another service adopting its use, and also interest from educators in ensuring that it was a valid tool. This resulted in me engaging in a formal period of research to investigate the validity and clinical utility of MOTOM, as part of a Masters of Philosophy. Further evaluation and development of MOTOM undertaken as part of this study included the following.

## Survey of users of MOTOM

A questionnaire was used to survey the views and opinions of the 37 occupational therapists using MOTOM within two NHS Trust occupational therapy services. One of the services was Morriston Hospital, where the tool had been developed, and significant changes to the documentation used had already been undertaken to ensure that MOTOM was integrated with minimal additional documentation. The other service had more recently implemented MOTOM, and so it was being used in addition to existing documentation. The questionnaire was piloted with four occupational therapists who were not going to be available to participate in the study. Feedback from the pilot enabled improvements to be made to the wording of questions to ensure clarity and lack of ambiguity and subsequent revision of some questions. The revised questionnaire was then piloted. The aim of the questionnaire was to elicit the views of the occupational therapists using MOTOM regarding clinical utility and construct validity of the tool. Clinical utility relates to how user-friendly a measure is in relation to issues such as how long it takes to use, how clear the instructions are, the acceptability of the presentation, and how appropriate is it for use. . Validity addresses whether the measure accurately assesses what it intends to, so the survey of opinion aimed to establish whether the therapist considered the outcome correlated with their perceived outcome for the service user, and also addressed issues such as the sensitivity of the rating scale.

## Audit

In order to gather data to evaluate how the 37 occupational therapists were using MOTOM in practice, a sample of 220 completed record cards were audited, taking 10 records from 22 clinical teams. Evaluating text from the main body of the record, the initial assessment forms and the intervention/outcome forms, an objective demonstration of MOTOM in practice was obtained. The records were audited against a checklist based on departmental standards and criteria developed for the study. The audit aimed to evaluate the thoroughness of the assessment process in identifying relevant problems, evidence of the service user/carer's views, use of outcome codes, evaluation of importance weightings used, correct rating of problems and outcomes, correct calculation of outcome scores, and use of occupational performance terminology.

## Service user or therapist rating?

Although the decision had already been made for the therapists to rate ability, as part of the investigation into construct validity, it was important to explore the service user's perception of their problems, abilities and outcomes of occupational therapy intervention in order to assess whether MOTOM was really measuring what it proposed to. The perception of a sample of individual service users in relation to the rating of their ability both before and after intervention, and the importance of that particular activity was established. In addition, their opinion as to whether all relevant issues had been covered was investigated.

### Significant changes to MOTOM

As a result of findings from the above studies, along with literature reviews of occupational therapy philosophy and models, outcome measures and psychometric properties, further amendments were made to MOTOM:

* Development of a comprehensive guide to using MOTOM
* Measurement of change in occupational performance status only
* Cessation of the importance weighting
* The production of a single outcome calculated as the median of individual outcome scores
* A rating scale change from a 4- to a 5-point scale to increase the sensitivity and incorporate rating of risk

For me, the most significant change was that of measuring only a change in occupational performance. Earlier versions of MOTOM included problems relating to environment and performance skills in addition to pure occupational performance. This was indicative of the historical approach to practice, and the lack of confidence in professional identity. Surely, as an occupational therapy specific outcome measure, what we need to measure is the unique contribution of occupational therapists, which is the facilitation of a change in our service users' occupational functioning in order to improve health and well-being. Prior to this change, many therapists were documenting problems in terms of performance skills, for example, 'reduced flexion of hip', and 'reduced standing tolerance', or environmental barriers, such as 'steep steps at front door'. It took significant time and education for therapists to consider problems in terms of occupational performance and to consider performance skills and environment in terms of how they impact on occupational performance. For some therapists, this focus on occupational performance was perceived as being simplistic, with the fear that it would not be regarded as technically skilled compared with the contribution of other members of the team who worked to a medical model. Encouragement was given to incorporate the performance skill deficit or environmental limitation as the reason why the occupational performance was limited. Discussions with colleagues have since identified this to be an extremely useful tool to help explain to others why occupational therapists undertake a particular activity that may be perceived at a superficial level, but actually has a clinically reasoned basis. It has also been useful in demonstrating the purpose of undertaking specific activities with patients, evidencing their relevance to the service user as an individual and to their rehabilitation programme.

## Summary: where are we in 2011?

The occupational therapy service within Morriston Hospital has been affected by several organisational restructurings, and is now one component of a much larger occupational therapy service. The current climate within NHS Wales has become financially focused reflecting the current economic climate of the whole country. The impact of this has been the loss of some occupational therapy posts in order to meet cost improvement targets, and a drive to redesign services to operate within the decreasing financial envelope. The challenges facing the service are maintaining the quality of service provision whilst practitioners face an ever increasing caseload. It is becoming increasingly important to evidence outcome of intervention in order to justify ongoing financial investment, and to maintain service provision. It is important that the occupational therapy service is proactive in providing evidence to demonstrate the effectiveness of areas of practice. There is recognition that MOTOM requires research into reliability, and its use within other services across the country following the publication within the British Journal of Occupational Therapy (James and Corr 2004) may support further research. Future challenges are ensuring that the documentation used is fit for purpose. The redesign of services is resulting in the expansion of occupational therapy roles, and the adaptation of documentation to reflect this is essential.

Finally, we as individual therapists are now strongly able to reflect on the role of the Model of Adaptation through Occupation (Reed and Sanderson 1983, 1992, 1999) in our attempts to reason, carry out and evaluate our occupationally based interventions and will continue to do so.

## Acknowledgements

The authors would like to acknowledge the support of Dr Gail Boniface and Mary Gilbert of the Welsh School of Occupational Therapy during the development of the Model of Adaptation through Occupation in 1991. They would also like to acknowledge Dr Susan Corr for her support with the research into the validity and clinical utility of MOTOM and all the occupational therapy staff who participated in the study.

## References

Eakin, P. (1991) Occupational therapy in stroke rehabilitation: implications of research into therapy outcome. *British Journal of Occupational Therapy* 54, 326–328.

James, S. and Corr, S. (2004) Morriston occupational therapy outcome measure (MOTOM): measuring what matters. *British Journal of Occupational Therapy* 67, 210–216.

Kielhofner, G. (1985) *Health Through Occupation: Theory and Practice in Occupational Therapy*. Philadelphia: F.A. Davis.

Law, M., Polatajko, H. and Pollock, N. (1994) Pilot testing of the Canadian Occupational Performance Measure: clinical and measurement issues. *Canadian Journal of Occupational Therapy* 61, 191–197.

MacAvoy, E. (1991) The use of ADL indices by occupational therapists. *British Journal of Occupational Therapy* 54, 383–385.

Mahoney, F.I. and Barthel, D.W. (1965) Functional evaluation: the Barthel Index. *Maryland State Medical Journal* 14, 56–61.

Reed, K. (1984) *Models of Practice in Occupational Therapy*. Baltimore/London: Lippincott, Williams and Wilkins.

Reed, K. and Sanderson, S. (1983) *Concepts of Occupational Therapy*, 2nd edn. Baltimore: Lippincott, Williams and Wilkins.

Reed, K. and Sanderson, S. (1992) *Concepts of Occupational Therapy*, 3rd edn. Baltimore. Lippincott, Williams and Wilkins.

Reed, K. and Sanderson, S. (1999) *Concepts of Occupational Therapy*, 4th edn. Philadelpdia: Lippincott, Williams and Wilkins.

Toomey, M., Nicholson, D. and Carswell, A. (1995) The clinical utility of the Canadian Occupational Performance Measure. *Canadian Journal of Occupational Therapy* 62, 242–249.

Townsend, E., Stanton, S., Law, M., Polatajko, H., Baptiste, S., Thompson-Franson, T., Kramer, C., Swedlove, F., Brintnell, S. and Campanile, L. (1997) *Enabling Occupation: An Occupational Therapy Perspective*. Ottawa, ON: CAOT ACE.

Unsworth, C. (1993) The concept of function. *British Journal of Occupational Therapy* 56, 287–292.

Ward, G., Jagger, C. and Harper, W.M.H. (1996) The Canadian Occupational Performance Measure: what do users consider important? *British Journal of Therapy and Rehabilitation* 3, 448–452.

Waters, D. (1995) Recovering from a depressive episode using the Canadian Occupational Performance Measure. *Canadian Journal of Occupational Therapy* 62, 278–282.

## Further reading

James, S. and Corr, S. (2004) Morriston Occupational Therapy Outcome Measure (MOTOM): measuring what matters. *British Journal of Occupational Therapy* 67, 210–216.

## Chapter 8

# Using the Canadian Model of Occupational Performance to reconfigure an integrated occupational therapy service

*Siân Waygood, Margot Mason, Heather Hurst, Tamsin Fedden and Caroline Phelps*

---

**Key points**

* An occupational therapy professional model offers a corporate identity to an occupational therapy service
* To maintain the implementation of a model a steering group is required
* Using a model will result in a change in practice
* It is essential to involve staff in the process of implementing a model

---

## Introduction

In this chapter, we will outline how we introduced an occupational therapy professional model and the organisational changes we introduced, which shaped the model's implementation. In 2004, the occupational therapy services within the county of Gloucestershire were reconfigured. This brought occupational therapists from a range of diverse organisations with varying cultures, political imperatives, systems and processes together within one integrated (across health and social care) service. This integration of the disparate service areas highlighted the need to find a common language for occupational therapy. A language that was not a health or social framework, but embraced the unique attributes and contributions we, as occupational therapists, could offer to organisations and residents alike within the county. It was also deemed critical that any framework adopted did not favour any specific staff group and that it presented a consistent corporate identity to all stakeholders. We felt that an occupational therapy professional model could offer us such a language, and therefore, we chose to implement the Canadian Model of Occupational Performance (Townsend et al 2002), as we

---

*Using Occupational Therapy Theory in Practice*, First Edition. Edited by Gail Boniface and Alison Seymour.
© 2012 Blackwell Publishing Ltd. Published 2012 by Blackwell Publishing Ltd.

felt it would provide a unified occupation-focussed language that offered the opportunity to bring the service together, at this time of significant change. In implementing this model within the newly restructured service, some key areas for consideration were identified: consultation and staff involvement, working with colleagues in academia, the varying approaches to intervention utilised by a range of staff groups and the pivotal role of the steering group created to enable the model's development within the service. Another factor that influenced the process we engaged in was integration of the model within different organisational systems, with a variety of service user groups and multi-disciplinary teams. Whilst the successes related to adopting the model will be evaluated in this chapter, key challenges to its implementation will also be reviewed. These will all be considered in relation to management decisions taken to embed the model and its background theory within practice and to maintain it as a tool to ensure that theory and evidence underpin all aspects of service delivery.

Finally, the benefits of using an evidence-based, client-centred model with a validated outcome measure will be reviewed in relation to national directives such as Health Professions Council (HPC) registration (HPC 2007), Agenda for Change and advanced practitioner roles (DH 2004), alongside the Personalisation Agenda and Putting People First initiatives (DH 2007). Initially, the local context will be reviewed as the starting point of the journey to adopting a model in practice.

# The local context

### Continuing professional development needs

In 2002, a collaborative submission was made for funding to the local Workforce Development Confederation seeking a dedicated resource to enhance and promote robust clinical governance within occupational therapy services in Gloucestershire. The aim was to commission research to identify the continuing professional development (CPD) needs of therapists, to ensure their skills and competencies matched the needs of service users, employing organisations and the profession. Funding was successful and a piece of research was undertaken that resulted in the document 'Fit for The Future' (Hurst 2003) that advocated amongst a number of recommendations, development of an occupational therapy professional model in the county to promote evidence-based and scholarly practice.

### Local re-organisation

Whilst the recommendations from the research were under consideration, a significant re-organisation was in progress across the health community. Occupational therapists were employed by three different National Health Service (NHS) trusts and the local county council and responsible between them for acute and community hospitals, intermediate care, adult and children's social care. At the time of integration, the occupational therapy service had 300 staff in the region. Initially the three trusts covering both acute and community health services were reconfigured and following a period of consultation occupational therapy services delivering acute and community physical therapy provision became integrated into one service hosted by a local Primary Care Trust. Subsequently, a project commenced to further align occupational therapy services by amalgamating the existing health services with colleagues based in Social Services.

### Occupational therapy service integration

In October 2004, Gloucestershire occupational therapy services were integrated under Health Act Flexibilities, Section 31, latterly Section 75 (DH 2006). The aims of the service post-integration were to promote more joint working across health and social care sectors, improve service users' pathways across organisations with better resource management, and thus subsequently provide a more responsive service. The service aspired to have consistent structures to promote accountability and to provide greater opportunities for CPD and a more robust career structure. In addition, the vision was to enable delivery of 'Best Practice' maintaining and improving delivery both in the context of therapeutic interventions and in achieving organisational targets. We recognised that as well as requiring a consistent corporate approach, we needed to ensure that the views and expectations of service users were integrated into our new service development. Finally, commissioning organisations wanted assurance that there were robust governance arrangements in place to demonstrate the quality, efficacy and value for money being offered by the service. Ultimately, the goal was to enable the development of a service based on client-centred and evidence-based practice with a culture of learning, delivering high quality, occupationally focussed interventions in a timely and effective way to the population of the county.

### Staff engagement

Prior to and around the time of reorganisation, staff were invited to attend a series of workshops in the county. The sessions were led by a colleague from Cardiff University, and the aim of the workshops was to engage with all qualified and support staff to explore the theory and application of models in practice. The sessions sought staff feedback and preferences in relation to the use of a model within the county. More detail will follow in relation to these workshops and how we implemented the model in practice; however, some initial challenges should be noted. The majority of staff expressed a preference for adopting the Canadian Model of Occupation Performance (CMOP; Townsend et al 2002) and most embraced the opportunities offered by adopting a model in their clinical practice. Other staff were both resistant or ambiguous about using a model. In addition, some service areas raised particular challenges in relation to adopting a model, for example the specialist wheelchair assessment service and occupational therapists working in hand therapy settings (see Section 'Challenges with some service areas'). Hence, the need for a steering group to support implementation with enthusiasts and sceptics alike was acknowledged (see Section 'Creating a learning organisation').

### Challenges with some service areas

Occupational therapists from the specialist wheelchair service attended the workshops with their colleagues. However, it was noted that the service employed Physiotherapists, Rehabilitation Engineers and support staff and, therefore, the applicability of an occupational therapy professional model in this clinical setting was debated. It could be argued that within this specialism of wheelchair mobility and postural management, an occupational therapist completes a holistic occupation-focussed assessment, considering the individual's home and work environment, the person's cognitive and physical abilities and their spiritual and cultural influences. However, it was also recognised that as a small multi-disciplinary service, therapists often had to focus their role on mobility and specialist seating, with other factors being left to colleagues in community and hospital teams. In practice, a pragmatic view was taken not to use the model as it was acknowledged that to extend the role beyond core mobility and seating would negatively impact on timely access to the service, which was a high priority for service users. In the case of those working in hand therapy, there were mixed views; a minority saw themselves as providing specialist interventions in splinting and upper limb rehabilitation without considering the wider occupational context. However, ultimately the majority felt the treatment of their clients did and should incorporate consideration of the impact on all aspects of the individual's life. Consequently, all occupational therapists working in hand therapy decided it was appropriate to fully utilise the CMOP within their practice.

## Creating a learning organisation

Back in 2004, we recognised that in order to embed the theory we needed to keep enthusiasm and momentum going. We will now be looking at the practicalities of implementing the CMOP across such a broad service.

Whilst occupational therapy leaders and managers generally had an understanding about why we wanted to overtly use theory to underpin practice, there was recognition that for successful implementation, all staff needed to be included in the decision-making process and own the changes to practice being made. The desire to create a learning culture with engagement from all staff groups needed support to systems to help it to happen (Senge et al 1999). The question for us was from whom and how would these systems be developed? To be successfully implemented by the many different groups of staff, there needed to be a way of creating effective communication systems, networks and shared identity. We believed a partnership among ourselves, the clinicians and colleagues in academia could help us. We believed using a single model, the CMOP, with an associated outcome measure could support us in creating a shared vision in the new occupational therapy service. We felt that this would lead to improvement in occupational therapy competency, and in time, lead to improving opportunities for occupational therapists working in Gloucestershire. Links with Cardiff University already existed and our academic colleague was invited to work with us.

This desire to have a more theoretical underpinning to our practice meant it seemed sensible to engage with *academic* services at an early stage. To become a learning organisation, responsive to local needs, a partnership was vital to ensure our service had a sound evidence base and was up to date with theory. In turn, academia would be influenced by practice using workplace evidence to inform the development of the theory.

Our academic colleague suggested a series of workshops to look at theory, identify what models were and what a model might offer to practitioners. The universal message from these workshops was that the staff wanted a model that focussed clearly upon occupation, with an attached outcome measure, and did not necessitate learning a whole new language. This naturally led us towards the CMOP (Townsend et al 1997, 2002). The important message that managers wanted to convey, and integral to successful adoption of the CMOP, was for staff to feel involved in decisions being made. In our large organisation, working areas were separated by many miles and to a certain extent this meant people needed to go away and get on with it. However, we recognised that people needed to feel they owned the changes taking place and recognise why a model had been adopted. To achieve this, we acknowledged there was a need to steer and direct the embedding process through creating systems to communicate about what was actually happening in the different areas.

### The CMOP steering group

Initially enthusiasts were called upon to work in the localities and join a short-term steering group. One of the first decisions of the steering group was to buy work books (Townsend and Wright 1998) so all areas could spend time really getting to grips with the CMOP (Townsend et al 2002) and gaining a fuller understanding of using the model in practice. How this would be done was largely left up to the individual areas themselves. However, it soon became clear that some areas were being more successful at this than others. This is exemplified by champions in the acute hospitals, who produced a training package on the model's theory and use. It soon became clear through discussions taking place within the steering group that other areas were keen to use this or a similar package to help them. There was recognition that the training package was a good way of a team working together to strengthen understanding of the CMOP, share how it could be practically adopted in individual clinical areas and address any issues or concerns. The steering group quickly realised this sharing of knowledge simply would not have happened if the information had not been taken to a group *steering* the implementation of the CMOP. Additionally, decisions taken by the steering group were greatly influenced by an earlier experience in Gloucestershire of using the measure associated with the model (Fedden et al 1999), the Canadian Occupational Performance Measure (COPM; Law et al 1991, 1994, 1998, 2005). This introduction of the measure in the 1990s resulted in many positive outcomes, but in hindsight, as it was not implemented with an underpinning of theory or the philosophy of the model, it failed. Therefore, when from a very early stage there was pressure on the steering group to develop CMOP paperwork and to direct and tell the staff how to use the model, it made a decision to resist both of these pressures. This decision was taken for several reasons, namely the steering group wanted to ensure that we as occupational therapists were all clear that what we were doing was occupational therapy; we needed to be able to use the CMOP to understand and consider our practice and finally to ensure our practice was occupational and client centred, rather than paperwork driven. Despite this call for paperwork, there were also staff anxieties that the use of the CMOP could create even more documentation and queries about how the paperwork would fit into areas where multi-disciplinary notes were being used, all of which the steering group sought to allay.

During its development, the steering group has inevitably involved people who are interested in practice developments. Many heated discussions have occurred and all members of the group have found that their thinking about occupational therapy practice has developed and changed. Debate has included evaluating and reflecting on custom and practice of occupational therapy not just the CMOP. Thus, it soon became apparent that the steering group, far from being a short-term group, was essential for communicating information across a wide staff group on an ongoing basis.

## Change management

The steering group remains pivotal in encouraging staff to use the CMOP whilst being responsive to the challenges its use presents. Literature highlights that supervisory managers are influential and play an important part in the successful implementation of any change (Senge et al 1999). The steering group recognised their supervisory and influential role but did not want staff to feel the model was being imposed upon them, rather that each individual was an active member of the change process. In any staff group there is a range of experience, length of service and very importantly a spectrum of personalities who vary in their willingness to change. Some had not studied models or theory at college, some had, but had not used them in practice, others had up to date theoretical knowledge and a few had practical experience. Within this wealth of experience, some embraced the use of the model wholeheartedly, a few needed more encouragement and others were stubbornly set in their ways and did not see the need to use a model!

A key driver for our desire to create a learning culture was to strengthen our corporate identity; meaning we needed to help staff understand and participate in the change process. Negotiation, support and encouragement of staff were vital. Ultimately we wanted staff to understand and recognise the benefit for all stakeholders of the occupational therapists' overtly using a model in practice.

## Dissemination of information

The steering group discussed what resources were required to assist staff confidence and keep the momentum going. Communication and dissemination of up to date information had been criticised by some staff and so we recognised that we needed to engage both occupational therapists and the managers in the different organisations. The steering group identified that although there were pockets of keen occupational therapists, the development of the use of the model could slip because of the lack of support and encouragement from management and senior occupational therapists. It was recognised by the steering group that managers also needed support to maintain enthusiasm for the model within their individual teams. Thus issues, concerns and good practice were brought to the steering group meetings, and over time tools and materials were developed to help staff in the sharing of good work and solutions to issues and concerns.

### Recognising our roles as researchers

This sharing of good (and bad) things has been vital in helping us to be responsive to the different pressures, and drivers required to help us continue to develop and grow. In terms of the action research that was occurring (Boniface et al 2008), the steering group clearly equated with being the researchers and as such the group reflected upon actions taken and then suggested new ideas and plans. Professionally, we could see the benefits of having a clearer understanding of our own occupational therapy identity and the unique influence our role has within different working areas.

### Keeping momentum going

We wanted to continue the process of embedding the model and developing our corporate identity and realised that new staff, who had not been involved in the original decision to implement a model, needed to be informed of the process, understand how the work had evolved and become active users of the CMOP. The steering group realised that the nature of an occupational therapy workforce meant that staff would move posts, and new staff needed to be provided with some kind of introduction to the model. Thus the CMOP training was included in staff induction processes. The steering group itself has continued to have an important role in making decisions and recognising when staff need re-energising. Whilst membership of the steering group has changed over the years, it continues to represent all grades of staff importantly recognising that all staff groups needed to have a voice in the change process.

## Training opportunities and tools

Over the years, a number of key tools and opportunities have been created to help staff to remain engaged with the process and to create our learning organisation. These include the following.

### One-day refresher workshop

The benefits of this for the wider service have been described earlier. Initially the creation of a training package was the idea of the acute hospital occupational therapist steering group representative. She felt that the most effective way of embedding the CMOP into staff practice was to gather a small action group of 'champions' in her area and put together a training programme based upon the workbook and textbook (Townsend and Wright 1998). This training package was then amended and rolled out across the whole service. As the training was evaluated, we changed its name to workshop as there was a strong feeling it was not a training of staff in the use of the CMOP, but rather an opportunity to reflect on the occupational nature of their own practice and reinforce this via the model. The name change of the training to workshop was felt to be an important yet subtle way of reinforcing this message.

The workshop content has been altered over time, following feedback from participants and facilitators and now it provides time out of the work environment for new staff to be introduced to the CMOP and existing staff to reflect upon use of the model, clinical reasoning and refocusing upon occupation. The day stresses the significance of going back to the roots of occupation and the importance of being able to articulate what occupational therapy can offer to clients and colleagues. It encourages the occupational therapist to think about the wider occupational needs of the client, not just what they can do themselves within their work environment and also promotes signposting to other services and settings. Participants generally leave the day enthused, whilst recognising the challenge is to keep their learning and development going in the pressures of the workplace. Some of the comments received from the workshops were as follows:

> It's all coming together for me. It's starting to feel more natural and become easier to relate to practice. I am getting there slowly.

> I had no knowledge of the CMOP previously but feel confident enough to have a go.

### Manual

Recognising that some occupational therapists would want something more concrete to refer to if they were to be successful in using the model in practice, a manual was produced by the steering group (Boniface et al 2010) and was given to all registered staff members. It explains why Gloucestershire decided to use a model, defines what a model is, answers questions staff might have about using the CMOP and gives completed examples of paperwork with guidelines to help clinicians to understand how the model might assist them to capture their clinical reasoning. Whilst it was acknowledged the manual could be seen as a concrete tool, we as a steering group saw it as remaining dynamic, when reviewed regularly and altered to reflect the changes in thinking of the service.

### Supervision DVD

The steering group recognised that people learn in different ways (Knowles 1975), and for some, a visual method might be beneficial. Supervision was seen as a good way of helping staff to explore their clinical actions and reasoning and so to develop their own practice. It was also a good way of reinforcing the model in clinical practice. Therefore combining these two things, a supervision DVD was produced containing a number of scenarios to help explore individual practice. Three members of the steering group compiled eight scenarios involving two occupational therapists in role play with one being a supervisor and the other the supervisee. The scenarios covered a number of different client groups and found the supervisor trying to encourage the supervisee to be more client and occupationally focussed during the intervention, despite challenges this could present in practice with time limitations.

The DVD is used both as a tool to support the model and as a teaching aid. Accompanying guidelines were produced so each scenario could be examined and discussed in more depth and related to one's own practice. It was envisaged that this would be done using one scenario at a time, in small manageable chunks, in staff meetings or CPD sessions.

### Away days

These were held specifically to enthuse staff, encourage shared identity, address areas of concern and reinforce professional responsibility. The content and groups of staff attending the away days has varied over the years. The 'who' depended upon need at the time, but at all times the main focus was to support and encourage staff and to deal with issues as they occurred or to re-energise staff. We never lost sight of the importance of communication not only within our own profession but also with colleagues and managers of the host organisations. We wanted to encourage a cohesive vision within our integrated service. The use of supervision (and DVD), case discussion and reflection were highlighted as important actions for staff and service development. Each away day also prompted and encouraged the use of group CPD sessions and journal clubs for wider professional activities.

### Newsletters

The steering group reported progress and achievements in using the CMOP via a quarterly occupational therapy newsletter. Good practices were reported focussing upon the work that was taking place in the different localities. Each newsletter contained a list of steering group representatives and contact details. Identifying who was on the steering group was important in letting everyone know they had a way of communicating and influencing the use of the CMOP in practice. These newsletters also served as a gentle prompt to remind people of the reasoning behind using a model and the benefits.

### Conferences

Motivation was high within the steering group and we wanted to share our practice with others and learn what was happening in other parts of the country. In 2006, the steering group hosted the first of the two local conferences with keynote presentations by Professor Thelma Sumsion on client-centred practice. Places were offered to staff from within Gloucestershire to share their own practice and network with colleagues from other parts of the country. Presentations have also been made at a number of College of Occupational Therapists conferences to share the development of the CMOP within Gloucestershire and learn about practices in other geographical areas.

### The journey

This communication has been important for us to help us to appreciate the ongoing nature of embedding the CMOP into our practice and recognise that it has no end (nor should it!) both locally and nationally. Instead it reinforces our own learning and development as occupational therapists. Now over 7 years after starting to use the CMOP, we have come to realise that using a model is an evolving process that needs to be re-energised regularly; otherwise it simply becomes seen as an 'add on' to the job and an abstract process. Our previous experience, as described in the preceding text, has been of the waning of enthusiasm when trying to implement the outcome measure associated with the model (COPM) on its own. At that time we did not use it with the CMOP and now believe our lack of understanding of the accompanying theory meant we did not fully appreciate the benefits of using an occupational therapy professional model and so gave it up at the earliest opportunity. We did not want this to happen again.

## The interface of occupational therapy practice within the wider organisation

This section outlines the benefits and challenges we face whilst implementing the CMOP within the wider organisations within which occupational therapists work in Gloucestershire.

### Challenges and our vision

It has undoubtedly proved to be a challenge to create a corporate occupational therapy identity, both within the NHS and Social Services hosting organisations. However, at the time of integration, we believed that the amalgamation of occupational therapy services would enable:

- more joint working across health and social care sectors;
- better resource management, increased ability to plan services countywide;
- an improved management structure;
- development of working groups to deliver and improve performance in key areas;
- countywide overview of staffing and demand;
- countywide overview of performance targets; and
- a better structure for staff education and CPD and ultimately enable the development of a service based on client-centred theory.

The outcome would be an actively learning organisation using one model of practice across working environments, which would lead to improved standards and consistency; clarity about what occupational therapists are doing and why; a vocabulary to articulate professional action and maintenance of professional identity. We believed practice needed to inform theory and vice versa. Our desire to reconsider the occupational element in a very wide and diverse service was one of the reasons the journey began. Thus we hoped that the use of a model would assist managers and staff at ground level to articulate what occupational therapy is, to assist with re-shaping the service, to receive appropriate referrals, to shed or delegate assessments or tasks that do not need a qualified occupational therapist's skills.

### Articulating theory in practice

The client-centred nature of the CMOP resonates with current health and social care expectations of creating more person-centred care and services the theory helped to strengthen the staff group's understanding and use of occupation, and also enabled them to articulate their unique contribution to clients more clearly. Staff were asked to consider how they introduced themselves to clients, carers and other members of the multi-disciplinary team. Through using the CMOP, we felt that the occupational therapists could focus upon occupation, facilitate clients to engage in their valued occupations and demonstrate the professional identity of occupational therapy to a wider team and employing organisation.

### Client-centred practice

The model's central tenet of client centredness is crucially important in the current health and social care governmental agenda. For example, Putting People First (DH 2010) emphasises a focus on person-centred or client-centred practice. Thus, occupational therapists basing their practice within the CMOP are in tune with current governmental as well as organisational expectations. We also believe that endeavouring to be client centred by utilising the CMOP has helped us to become more effective workers across health and social care boundaries.

### Challenges within both health and social care settings

Using the model requires the occupational therapist in both settings not only to act in a client-centred way but also to consider all occupational areas, not just the ones that the organisation within which they work may wish them to concentrate on such as self-care. It also needs to be acknowledged that time and resources can be limited so that the occupational therapist cannot always provide solutions across all occupational areas, but their identification via the model means that the occupational therapist can endeavour to give information or signpost the client on to other services. Supervision, ongoing learning and management support are crucial to assist therapists to fully use the model and not be overly influenced by organisational pressures. An example would be in using client-centred documentation but playing lip service to it, and not actually completing a client-centred assessment.

## Documentation

When utilising the model, all paperwork not only needs to overtly support client-centred practice and address all occupational areas but also address and conform to the organisational processes. The core message from the steering group to staff is to demonstrate quality clinical reasoning and overt use of the model in whatever documentation they use. This information should be clearly understood by other professionals. Gloucestershire developed different documentation across health and social care prior to integration, and since. The different organisations' electronic recording systems also made it difficult to share information. In Gloucestershire's experience, CMOP is easily useable in that it can both slot into existing generic documentation and create specific CMOP-orientated documentation. In health, although specific CMOP-orientated documentation has been designed successfully, there have been issues around where this is recorded and duplication of information needed, for example in nursing notes on the wards. In Social Care, staff have used the generic documentation effectively through using the headings of the model when compiling assessments. Powerfully this helped the occupational therapist to focus upon being occupationally focussed rather than problem orientated. Although initially seen as a compromise it has worked well as it is an electronic system so documents are accessible to all professionals involved. Developments continue and an occupational therapy professional assessment has been developed to run alongside the generic information gathering tools. At a team level, understanding of occupational therapy has improved. The use of CMOP has encouraged a dialogue between professionals and increased clarity of role. However, there have been difficulties in some multi-disciplinary settings with fear of change from occupational therapy staff and others. Some occupational therapists, colleagues and managers saw CMOP documentation as increasing the workload. In certain areas, the use of multi-disciplinary goal setting has proved a challenge to documenting their use of the model. Again, this has been seen as a challenge because using the model forms an overt change to practice. Whether documentation is separate or joint, occupational therapists' recording should clearly show their clinical reasoning and occupational focus in a proportionate manner, that is recording short, succinct and occupationally based assessments and interventions.

Initially when implementing the CMOP we believed that we would be using the associated outcome measure COPM fairly quickly. However, our experiences have shown how important it has been to embed the understanding of the model first. Within such a large staff group, this has taken over 7 years to encourage joined up working and shared identity. We are now at the stage of implementing the COPM as our outcome measure. We believe that the COPM is an ideal tool to capture client satisfaction and we are looking forward to seeing the benefits of using it for the client, occupational therapist, employing organisation and profession as a whole.

## Conclusion

Reflecting on introducing a model across a range of diverse and newly integrated occupational therapy services not only highlights the significant barriers encountered but also the many benefits to practice. From a management perspective, the process of embedding a model to underpin practice is time-consuming and requires both ongoing work and a varied approach to ensure that staff remain engaged and committed to its use within all work settings. The steering group was critical in guiding the model's implementation and in sustaining motivation and energy across the service. The group also became the centre of philosophical and pragmatic discussions in relation to questions that challenged historical custom and practice. The process of implementing the use of a model, like any change process, is lengthy and undoubtedly requires support from leaders, but equally or even more important, are 'Champions' from within the service – from all levels, as these clinicians not only offer guidance to peers but also challenge colleagues far more convincingly than directives from managers, and their influence should not be underestimated.

Utilising theory has engendered debate and discussion and has often led to vigorous and healthy questioning in many areas of service delivery. The model has clarified the role of professionally qualified staff and the very experienced and knowledgeable support staff that combine to ensure the most effective teams. All aspects of clinical provision have been explored, including the traditional roles that therapists have been identified with; that is the discharge therapist or the person that provides equipment. The model has ensured reflection regarding the most appropriate skill mix to meet clients' needs and this has, on occasions, meant relinquishing roles to other health professionals and support staff as it has been recognised that they are not core occupationally focussed interventions.

The adoption of a client-centred, evidence-based occupational therapy professional model with a validated outcome measure has proven to be in synergy with a range of current national developments. The introduction of HPC registration has been timely, as the emphasis on scholarly practices with explicit occupation and outcome-focused clinical interventions provides the staff with readily available and overt evidence of competence and CPD. The development of the Personalisation Agenda and 'Putting People First' initiative (2007) is consistent and synonymous with client-centred practice so the service is well placed to demonstrate and contribute to delivering organisational targets. The quality and outcome measures required by the organisation can readily be evidenced and supported by the use of the model and consequently the service is well prepared to meet the future challenges, both professionally and in support of our wider-commissioning organisations. For our service users, the utilisation of the model puts them at the heart of any intervention; coupled with the fact that the outcome measure can provide feedback on the efficacy of service delivery and the appropriateness of the services interventions, thus promoting the best and most effective use of resources to meet their needs. Finally, we firmly believe that using the CMOP has helped us to be responsive to the requirements of both the local drivers (employing organisations) and the statutory agencies (HPC and COT).

# References

Boniface, G, Fedden, T., Hurst, H., Mason, M., Phelps, C., Reagon, C. and Waygood, S. (2008) Using theory to underpin an integrated occupational therapy service through the Canadian Model of Occupational Performance. *British Journal of Occupational Therapy* 71(12), 531–539.

Boniface, G., Hurst, H. and Waygood, S. (2010) *A Gloucestershire Interpretation for Implementing the Canadian Model of Occupational Performance in a UK Setting: A Users Guide.* Cardiff: Cardiff University.

Department of Health (DH) (2004) *Agenda for Change.* Leeds:  DH.

Department of Health (2006) *NHS Act 2006 Partnership Arrangements.* Leeds: DH.

Department of Health (2007) *Putting People First: A Shared Vision and Commitment to the Transformation of Adult Social Care.* Leeds: DH.

Department of Health (2010) *Prioritising Need in the Context of Putting People First: A Whole System Approach to Eligibility for Social Care. Guidance on Eligibility Criteria for Adult Social Care.* Leeds: DH.

Fedden, T., Green, A. and Hill, T. (1999) Out of the woods, the Canadian Occupational Performance Measure from the Manual to Practice. *British Journal of Occupational Therapy* 62(7), 318–320.

Health Professions Council (HPC) (2007) *Standards of Proficiency – Occupational Therapists.* London: HPC.

Hurst, H. (2003) *Fit for the Future Strategy Document.* Gloucester: West Gloucestershire Primary Care Trust and Gloucestershire Social Services.

Knowles, M.S. (1975) *Self-Directed Learning: A Guide for Learners and Teachers.* Englewood Cliffs, NJ: Prentice Hall.

Law, M., Baptiste, S., Carswell, A., McColl, M., Polatajko, H. and Pollock, N. (1991) *Canadian Occupational Performance Measure.* Toronto: CAOT Publications.

Law, M., Baptiste, S., Carswell, A., McColl, M., Polatajko, H. and Pollock, N. (1994) *Canadian Occupational Performance Measure*, 2nd edn. Toronto: CAOT Publications.

Law, M., Baptiste, S., Carswell, A., McColl, M., Polatajko, H. and Pollock, N. (1998) *Canadian Occupational Performance Measure*, 3rd edn. Ottawa, ON: CAOT ACE.

Law, M., Baptiste, S., Carswell, A., McColl, M., Polatajko, H. and Pollock, N. (2005) *Canadian Occupational Performance Measure*, 4th edn. Ottawa, ON: CAOT ACE.

Senge, P., Kleiner, A., Roberts, C., Ross, R., Roth, G. and Smith, B. (1999) *The Dance of Change: The Challenges of Sustaining Momentum in Learning Organizations The Challenges of Sustaining Change in Learning Organizations (A Fifth Discipline Resource).* New York: Doubleday.

Townsend, E. and Wright, W.A. (1998) *Enabling Occupation: A Learner-Centred Workbook.* Ottawa, ON: CAOT ACE.

Townsend, E., Stanton, S., Law, M., Polatajko, H., Baptiste, S., Thompson-Franson, T., Kramer, C., Swedlove, F., Brintnell, S. and Campanile, L. (1997) *Enabling Occupation: An Occupational Therapy Perspective*. Ottawa, ON: CAOT ACE.

Townsend, E., Stanton, S., Law, M., Polatjko, H., Baptiste, S., Thompson-Franson, T., Kramer, C., Sedlove, F., Brintnell, S. and Campanile L. (2002) *Enabling Occupation: An Occupational Therapy Perspective*, 2nd edn. Ottawa, ON: CAOT ACE.

## Further reading

Boniface, G., Fedden, T., Hurst, H., Mason, M., Phelps, C., Reagon, C. and Waygood, S. (2008) Using theory to underpin an Integrated Occupational Therapy Service through the Canadian Model of Occupational Performance. *British Journal of Occupational Therapy* 71(12), 531–539.

## Chapter 9

# Dealing with the barriers to change whilst implementing the Canadian Model of Occupational Performance

*Jane Walker and Gillian Thistlewood*

---

**Key points**

- Implementing a model requires the use of champions and a bottom-up approach
- The model's theory needs to be embedded across all processes in which the occupational therapists engage
- Implementing a model within a multi-disciplinary setting requires good communication
- There needs to be an identifiable differentiation between the roles of registered occupational therapists and support staff

---

## Introduction

In this chapter, we discuss the issues, decisions and barriers we encountered when attempting to implement the Canadian Model of Occupational Performance (CMOP) within the occupational therapy service across National Health Service (NHS), Gloucestershire. CMOP (Townsend et al 2002) was introduced in Gloucestershire in 2004, following the outcome of a research study that identified the need for a common theoretical framework across the service (see Chapter 8) (Hurst 2003). With the support of a countywide steering group, local champions were instrumental in the successful implementation of the model's theory through enabling the development of training, documentation and peer review. The champions, via local sub-groups, challenged peer thinking on clinical reasoning and encouraged confident application of the model within practice. In addition, formal training enhanced knowledge and professional confidence in articulating occupational therapy theory and practice to others within the multi-disciplinary team (MDT).

As a consequence of introducing theory to practice, discussions ensued regarding the distinction between the roles and responsibilities of registered occupational therapists compared to support workers engaged in delivering occupational therapy. Consequently, a delegation framework was formulated based on professional experience and reflection.

---

*Using Occupational Therapy Theory in Practice*, First Edition. Edited by Gail Boniface and Alison Seymour.
© 2012 Blackwell Publishing Ltd. Published 2012 by Blackwell Publishing Ltd.

This framework was subsequently introduced to all service areas to guide and support the decision-making process, regarding the appropriate delegation of work.

In this chapter, therefore, we discuss the process of implementing the model and the consequential delegation framework and it is hoped that this discussion will enable readers to gain a greater understanding of the challenges encountered when introducing a theoretical framework into established working practice. Uncovering the challenges for us identified several influencing factors including organisational, individual, inter-professional teamwork and practice issues, which we intend to discuss here.

## The challenge of working with an organisation

Implementing new ways of working, within any organisation, requires staff and key stakeholders to engage in a process of change. The journey requires a sense of vision. Breaking down barriers to understanding professional roles can be made clearer with a framework to support operational delivery. It can provide a common language, identity and stronger partnerships in delivering client-centred practice. Some key challenges encountered in model implementation in organisations will now be discussed.

### The organisational climate

In the United Kingdom, the political climate supports client-centred practice, as indicated in the National Service Framework for Older People (Department of Health 2001). This sets standards for good practice and aims to ensure that older people are treated as individuals and enabled to make choices (Department of Health 2001). However, both Nocon and Pleace (1998) and Awang (2002) evidenced a lack of client-centred practice by occupational therapists within social care settings, highlighting issues such as a lack of client involvement in the decision-making process, poor grant publicity and lack of democratic control for service users. Therapists may perceive that they work in a client-centred way, but without a full understanding of the challenges and complexities of what this means in practice. In social care, the risk of being partially client-centred is increased due to the complex legal framework, eligibility criteria and performance indicators. Within health care, bed pressures create a demand for clear decision-making on client needs for discharge, in shorter timeframes. Occupational therapists are working with organisations that exist to meet the health needs of a population, and bed turnover and targets are required to achieve this. Duty of care needs to be explicitly understood by services accepting referrals and passing on unmet needs, which are often complex in nature. Additionally, such occupational therapists need to be supported to accept the boundaries of their intervention and need to discharge duty of care effectively.

Organisational challenges will continue, but maintaining professional identity within a framework, as well as understanding the organisational pressures, is a key role in professional leadership.

## Promoting the ethos of a model

Therapists and their support staff are key, at an operational level, in promoting the ethos and principles of the framework and client-centred practice. In the first author's (Walker 2008) MSc study carried out with staff within NHS Gloucestershire occupational therapy services, the difficulty of ensuring continuity of approach whilst using the model was identified. Since re-organisation (see Chapter 8), a sense of fragmentation remained, as well as lack of a cohesive structure. Some therapists felt that the model should bring unity across the integrated occupational therapy service and looked to the steering group (see Chapter 8) to ensure the model was embedded in practice and its development was supported. This group challenged attitude, knowledge and resource development, across health and social care, which enabled barriers to be worked on.

When implementing a model in practice, it is important to ensure there is a flow of communication of information. Ideas on how to implement the model and overcome barriers, as well as progress in different service areas should be shared. Furthermore, cascading of information regarding the overall progress of theory implementation is also important, as well as information from the steering group members, supplementary written information on a regular basis may be of value. Implementing regular documentation audits to evaluate the appropriate use of the framework is important. Audit results need to be communicated to individuals to enable improvement in key areas.

Embedding a process of evaluation in terms of implementation is vital. This was demonstrated by Deegan et al's (2005) study that highlighted the need for regular evaluation and audit to help to ensure that the change process continues and can then be transferred to other areas of practice.

## Recruiting and retaining staff

In Gloucestershire, the model was embedded in recruitment and retention strategies within the organisation from initial implementation stages. This included a review of all advertising, promotional materials and job descriptions, which depending on the post, include awareness, knowledge or practical experience in using the CMOP (Townsend et al 2002). Existing staff were supported in their continuing professional development for their role as well as to meet the Health Professions Council registration requirements (HPC 2007). This was done via reflection on the model at supervision, by case review, focusing on their use of the model in work settings and with individual client groups. Annual appraisal, using the NHS Knowledge and Skills Framework (Department of Health 2004), was another tool, which was used to identify key objectives and learning needs for each staff member, related to the use of the model. Leaders in the organisation were encouraged to strongly emphasise the ethos of client-centred practice, being key to occupational therapy and attracting and retaining the right staff to deliver this.

## Professional documentation

Professional documentation should be a tool, which clearly evidences clinical reasoning, the assessment process, intervention plan and outcome for each client. When implementing a model (see Chapter 8 for the reasoning behind this), it was decided at an early stage of implementation that specific paperwork should not be introduced until the theoretical context was fully understood. Prior to the implementation of the model, it was evident that recording methods varied according to the setting and were not standardised or evidenced based. As implementation progressed, professional documentation that clearly demonstrates clinical reasoning and application of the model was created.

In some settings, there may be a pressure to create generic assessments and one health care record to minimise the number of records held on one client by various departments. Translating the model, as a professional framework, into inter-disciplinary working creates challenges in terms of understanding and use (see Section 'The challenge of working with individuals' for further discussion on this). In other settings, such as social care, there may be existing documentation, which is recorded electronically. The use of a generic overview assessment in social care, which was not profession specific, failed to support the application of a model in professional practice. However, although the generic form was not universally liked by occupational therapists, it had become familiar and could be completed easily by individuals due to its familiarity. Due to the challenges of changing the electronic systems within social care settings, initial professional summaries were adapted by framing them to demonstrate clinical reasoning via the model's headings. Lack of a defined specific assessment or professional documentation can be frustrating for staff and may prevent moving forward with the implementation of a framework such as an occupational therapy professional model. Consequently, staff may need support to meet the organisational and the professional recording requirements and to identify a pragmatic, profession-specific way of recording their actions.

In contrast, within an acute hospital setting, the therapists had autonomy to design and introduce a profession-specific assessment form that was based on the model. However, even this was not without its challenges. Some occupational therapists found that the six sheets of the CMOP assessment, which was consequently created, were very lengthy to complete compared with their previous one-page assessment form. However, generally, the introduction of a CMOP assessment form provided a clear occupationally based structure for recording and made it easier to become familiar with the model and its concepts. Whatever the challenges of creating model-based documentation, it would appear to be important in order for staff to base their theory in something as concrete as an assessment and recording form that reflects the theory. However, the desire for paperwork must not be allowed to overtake the need to understand the concepts such paperwork uses and this was why the steering group (see Chapter 8) had initially been reluctant to create documentation forms before staff had begun to understand the concepts behind such paperwork (see also Chapter 6). The consequences of this decision were that the paperwork was created by the staff group, not by the steering group, and a bottom-up approach to change was apparent. This need to somehow get right and streamline documentation when introducing a practice model has also been highlighted by Bachman and Malloch (1998), who emphasised the lack of response and interest of practitioners in a model, prior to the revision of existing documentation.

With cases transferring across providers, a shared view on documentation may offer value. In Gloucestershire, using a CMOP assessment form was found to be useful initially in assisting understanding and guiding the occupational therapist through the application of the model. It also appeared to assist with communication from one occupational therapist to the next, where caseloads were shared, even across settings. However, as staff became more familiar with the model and understood the concepts, they tended to prefer the freedom of using the model less rigidly, following more of a free flowing format, especially within social care. Therefore, there is a necessity and flexibility for experienced practitioners to have the autonomy to use and apply the model in the way that they choose.

## The challenge of working with individuals

In the first author's previously mentioned study, factors relating to individual occupational therapists appear to present a significant challenge to the use of the CMOP. These include prior experience of practice models, opportunities for knowledge acquisition and attitudinal factors.

Lack of understanding of the concepts and application of the CMOP can greatly impact on its use by individual therapists. Additionally, those who have been practising for many years may be apprehensive regarding its introduction. Some find the language complicated and initially struggle to gain a full understanding of the model, whilst others express particular difficulties with the concept of spirituality. Although consideration of spirituality is perceived to be essential to CMOP, with its emphasis on holistic and client-centred practice, the potential confusion caused by the concept has previously been highlighted by many (Taylor et al 2000; Clarke 2003; Egan and Swedersky 2003; Beagan and Kumas-Tan 2005; Hoyland and Mayers 2005).

In order to facilitate knowledge and understanding of the CMOP, occupational therapists need to access a range of learning and development opportunities, some of which are more effective than others. As there was no training commercially available, occupational therapists based within the acute hospital designed and delivered a comprehensive training package, which appeared to be very useful in assisting their understanding of the CMOP. Furthermore, understanding of the CMOP appears to correlate with motivation to use the model. By contrast, occupational therapists within community settings suggested that the roll out of the CMOP appeared to flounder at the start. Some occupational therapists suggest that the initial lack of formal training in some areas of the county was a significant factor that had contributed to variations in use by individual therapists.

Recognition has been given to the importance of maintaining and building on the enthusiasm initially generated in order to ensure that the momentum is not lost. The presence of a countywide steering group comprising representatives or *champions* from each area is significant in sustaining the pace of change. The enthusiasm and skills of the champions is vital in providing the link between the theory and practical utility of the model. Theoretical knowledge in isolation is not sufficient to ensure the integration of a model in practice. Formal training has to be supplemented by regular practical sessions, during which occupational therapists have the opportunity to discuss case examples and debate practice issues within their regular intervention area.

These themes had also been highlighted by Warren (2002) previously, concluding that training that encompasses both the philosophy of the CMOP and its practical utility are essential if it is to be successfully applied in practice. Similarly, the importance of staff education time, when encouraging the use of client-centred theory, such as the CMOP, has been emphasised (Sumsion and Smyth 2000). The significance of an identifiable person or a group who is responsible for the change process involved when moving towards a client-centred approach is also important (Wilkins et al 2001). The use of case studies and sharing ideas amongst therapists have also been suggested as a potential solution to challenging such practice issues (Sumsion and Smyth 2000; Wilkins et al 2001).

### Attitude

The attitude of individual therapists to the introduction of the CMOP varies considerably and appears to be influenced by their previous knowledge and experience of models in general and the CMOP in particular. The most recent graduate occupational therapists appeared to be excited by the idea and embraced it with enthusiasm. By contrast, experienced practitioners may be apprehensive about the introduction of new ideas and concepts with which they are unfamiliar. The necessity to embrace attitudinal change when introducing a new model has been observed and highlighted by previous authors (Bachman and Malloch 1998; Devine and Hirsh 1998; Lester 1998; Buchanan-Barker 2004; Hannigan 2004; Deegan et al 2005; Jeris et al 2008). These studies clearly highlight the importance of human factors during change initiation and emphasise the risks of neglecting these. In addition, there appears to be a difference in the perceived value of the CMOP by individuals, which once again seems to be linked to the length of postgraduate experience of practitioners. The perception of experienced practitioners is sometimes that the CMOP is more beneficial to new graduates in order to provide structure and guidance in their practice. Experienced graduates often perceive that their skills and experience as an occupational therapist, including their clinical reasoning, are already well-developed and refined, and therefore, the model offers only limited benefit. Thus, ignoring attitudes to change could have resulted in a staff-based perception that the model was only applicable in certain settings and to certain staff.

Part of the reason for adopting an occupational therapy professional model is to challenge the practice of the individual in order to make it more client-centred and less organisationally led. However, the introduction of a model can be perceived by some individuals to simply require a change to recording their practice rather than an actual change to their practice and intervention. Alternatively, occupational therapists who are reluctant to change their practice may already be practising in a client-centred way, rather than having failed to grasp the client-centred central concept of the CMOP (Towsend et al 2002). Whichever possibility is the case, the client-centred and occupational nature or occupational therapy practice needs to be articulated and the structured nature of the model can assist in this articulation. For example, occupational therapists within social care settings are employed to meet the statutory requirements of the Local Authority. Traditionally, the pressure of waiting lists and expectation of equipment provision has reinforced the limited perception of the role of the occupational therapist in this practice setting (Mountain 2000). Consequently and without the support of the model, some occupational therapists have been poor at supporting people with aspects of living with and adapting to disability and supporting their wider psychosocial needs (Mountain 2000). Similarly, Wilcock (2003) claimed that many practitioners have neglected to address the individual's range of occupational needs. Thus, the drive for fast discharge from hospital and preventing unnecessary hospital admissions have resulted in a lack of attention to wider issues such as vocational, social and creative needs of the individual. Wilcock (2003) suggested that the profession needed to be true to its own values but acknowledged the difficulties of this when others in the team are in a position of power and impose their requirements upon the occupational therapist.

The view of some therapists of the nature of client centredness has previously been observed by Wilkins et al (2001). Therapists can regard this approach as being something that they have always adopted and, therefore, fail to see the need to change (Wilkins et al 2001). Thus, occupational therapists adopting a client-centred approach require enhanced skills to ensure that it is effectively integrated into practice and visible (Wilkins et al 2001). Such therapists require role models, support and supervision to ensure that a client-centred approach is fully embraced and adopted in practice.

## The challenge of working in an inter-professional team

In addition to individual factors, team factors play an important role in the use of CMOP by individual therapists. Significant factors include the team structure and the impact of multi-disciplinary working.

### Team structure

The first author's study identified that the skill mix within some teams, with the inclusion of both new graduates, students and more experienced practitioners, appears to have a positive effect upon the use of the CMOP, as the students and newer graduates bring their enthusiasm and understanding to the team. In addition, occupational therapists describe the knowledge, experience and leadership qualities of the immediate line manager as being significant. The importance of a participatory management style has previously been highlighted by Wilkins et al (2001), who concluded that it was the most important factor in determining satisfaction during change initiation. Moreover, this style of management is believed to promote the sharing of ideas and prioritisation of changes essential to facilitate the change process (Wilkins et al 2001). Mullins (2005) also emphasised the necessity of co-operation between managers and staff members during the successful implementation of new working practices.

Although occupational therapists did not necessarily share the same initial enthusiasm, knowledge or experience, there appeared to be value in shared working and support within teams. A cohesive team, comprising an appropriate combination of skills and abilities, combined with a supportive manager, who is able to lead and encourage the team members, appears to facilitate the use of the CMOP by the individual team members due to shared experience and supportive working practices.

### Multi-disciplinary team working

Various issues present significant challenges to using the CMOP within an MDT. Some of these arise when recording assessments and interventions, whilst others relate to (sometimes entrenched) attitudes and perceptions of other professional groups.

Some occupational therapists are required to record their interventions within multi-disciplinary formats, which appears to present difficulties, mostly because they are obliged to record their intervention in several places. Previous studies have also concluded that some therapists found it very time consuming to complete a specific CMOP assessment form in addition to a more generic team assessment record (Warren 2002).

In addition, some occupational therapists feel obliged to modify their recording for the MDT, due to the team's lack of understanding of the concepts contained within the CMOP. Some suggest that using occupational therapy specific terminology could present a barrier to communication within the MDT. Potentially, modification of the language of the CMOP could compromise the use of this model, which advocates the application of a shared philosophy and language. Previous research studies concluded that the CMOP can assist the therapist to be able to articulate the theory behind their practice rather than allowing others to define their role and intervention (Warren 2002; Clarke 2003). By avoiding the language of occupation, therapists may fail to take advantage of the opportunity to educate others about the extent and purpose of occupational therapy intervention, thus negating one of the most important benefits of applying a practice model and reinforcing others misperceptions regarding occupational therapy practice and intervention.

In addition, occupational therapists raise issues relating to the expectations of other MDT members with regard to the occupational therapy role and intervention. This is particularly significant for occupational therapists working within a hospital-based environment, where the expectations of the whole MDT team are focused on the early discharge of the patient. Occupational therapists within hospital settings seem to be much more aware of the expectations of other MDT members and this appears to put them under pressure to conform to the roles and interventions desired by others. Some occupational therapists have to spend quite a lot of their time within the hospital setting, justifying their use of the CMOP. Nursing staff can be perceived as being very *task-orientated* and, therefore, asking the patient what is important to them could be seen as irrelevant (Walker 2008). By contrast, another occupational therapist in the first author's study (Walker 2008) described how the use of CMOP had actually improved her rapport with the physiotherapists within her team.

Thus, it would appear that the level of professional respect that exists between different professionals varies within the hospital setting. Previous research findings suggest that the CMOP may be difficult to apply in workplace settings dominated by the medical model (Clarke 2003; Sumsion and Smyth 2000). The traditional view, outlined in the medical model, is based on technical and scientific knowledge and is in direct contrast with one of the key concepts of the CMOP, which is concerned with the individual and the concept of client-centred practice. Moreover, the values epitomised within the CMOP are ideologically separate from the medical model, thus presenting challenges for occupational therapists as they try to implement the principles in a setting where their core values are misunderstood and misinterpreted.

Interestingly, the occupational therapists working within social care community teams describe a very different experience of MDT working. Some occupational therapists feel that their social care colleagues were probably not even aware of the introduction of the CMOP and could not see why it should have an impact on anyone else. By contrast, others have received positive feedback from their MDT colleagues regarding their CMOP-based assessments and recording, as they found that they were easy to read, provided comprehensive information and provoked discussion within the MDT. This could be explained by the view that occupational therapy has a great deal in common with social work, as social work also advocates the need to empower people to retain control over their lives (Thompson 2002). Thus, the misconceptions regarding the role of the occupational therapist are not as evident within the community teams as within the hospital setting.

Previous researchers advocate the advantages of using the CMOP to enable therapists to articulate their role more effectively, thus facilitating effective multi-disciplinary working, service evaluation and development (Warren 2002; Clarke 2003). In addition, it can provide a professional identity and clarify the role of the occupational therapist (Warren 2002). However, other study findings suggest that all staff within a team should be involved in client-centred training, as it can be difficult for some individuals within a team to adopt this approach whilst others have not (Sumsion and Smyth 2000). Thus, the culture of the organisation or service unit must support client-centred values in order to facilitate its use by individuals (Mortenson and Dyck 2006) and using the CMOP can influence this.

## The challenges of using theory in professional practice

The second author of this chapter has spent some time considering the practical challenges within Gloucestershire presented by using the model across a range of physical settings. These were related to both professional practice and service delivery. It is accepted that the model underpins the need to deliver client-centred, occupational-focused and evidence-based practice. However, in a changing health and social care system, application of these principles can be challenging for practitioners and managers. These challenges can be particularly pertinent when considering the involvement in the use of theory of a profession by its support workers or even more generic support workers.

## Delegation

The model clearly defines the role of the qualified therapist, but there was a need to include support workers, as part of the skill mix, in supporting client needs and effective service delivery. The risk of occupational therapists using merely technical skills is that these are devalued by others and perceived as not requiring a registered occupational therapist (Feaver and Creek 1993). In exploring how case and task allocation were handled by occupational therapists, several challenges arose, which were reflected in the following comments:

> The Occupational Therapy technician has worked here for 10 years and is really good at her job, so does it matter if she does a bit of occupational therapy?
>
> (An occupational therapist)

> I could support 2 occupational therapy assistants with the money allocated to that project for the cost of one occupational therapist – would mean I get more staff for the same money.
>
> (An NHS Primary Care Trust locality manager)

> Cover for the occupational therapist's annual leave is sorted, the occupational therapy technician will cover the ward.
>
> (An occupational therapist)

As funding within government services becomes ever pressurised, there is a need to clearly define the variances in levels of worker to meet client needs. Therapists feel pressure to continue to maintain cover for their clinical area during absence. Yet, managers and possibly clients demand professional accountability and the right skill mix to meet the right need. There are distinct differences in qualified staff and support workers, but together, there could be a unique combination of different skills equally valued, which can assist in embedding a model in practice. To understand the variation in practice and understanding of theory use between registered and support staff, a review of delegation within occupational therapy was undertaken with some training to support competence. The review's conclusion firstly defined two terms, *delegation* and *assignment*, based on ideas contained within the Intercollegiate Information Paper (CSP et al 2006):

* *Delegation* is the process by which a registered practitioner can allocate work to a support worker who is deemed competent to undertake that task. This worker then carries the responsibility for that task, while the registered practitioner retains accountability. The worker within Occupational Therapy, who can accept delegated cases, would be referred to as a support worker higher level or a technician.

- *Assignment* applies when both the responsibility and accountability for an activity passes from one individual to another.

Choosing tasks or roles to be undertaken by support staff is a complex professional activity. It is important to consider the competence of the support worker in relation to the activity to be delegated. Thus, the kind of comments that began this section need to be challenged in order to justify the differences between registered qualified and support staff.

In using the CMOP and CMOP-E (Townsend et al 2002; Townsend and Polatajko 2007), the registered practitioner must ensure that delegation or assignment of cases is appropriate in terms of client need and competence of the support worker. Clients who have complex occupational performance needs, which may require a spectrum of approaches, should be allocated to a qualified therapist who will have developed a range of assessment and intervention skills as part of their education.

However, if the client is likely to have a predictable care pathway that will require a straightforward technician type problem-solving approach, these cases can be assigned to support staff with the relevant skills.

Several clinical areas reviewed delegation within their teams. For oncology and palliative care in acute and community settings, staff reviewed caseloads to enable a clearer definition of simple and complex cases, which would enable them to complete and audit assignments of cases consistently. Although, designed for the oncology and palliative care specialist area as described in the preceding text, the examples mentioned later could be applied or adapted to a range of other areas and used to review the relationship between qualified staff and support workers' roles. The examples are as follows:

*Simple case*: It describes a predictable pathway, which will be suitable to assign to a support worker and may include the following situations:

- Where the patient is able to participate in and understand therapy intervention and has minimal cognitive, emotional or communication problems.
- Where the patient has a stable and consistent level of social support.
- Where the patient is mobile with/without use of equipment or with the help/ supervision of one person.
- Where few problems anticipated in the fields of personal care or kitchen, if these assessments are considered necessary.
- Where the patient lives in accessible accommodation or sheltered housing.
- Where few problems are anticipated for the delivery/fitting and demonstration of use of equipment for home use.
- Where prior to a support worker completing community visits, there had been established contact and communication between the occupational therapy team with patient's family/carers, prior to discharge.
- Where an unproblematic and predictable discharge from hospital/hospice is anticipated/completed.
- Where a predictable rehabilitation pathway is expected to be needed post-discharge.

*Complex case*: It describes an unpredictable pathway, which will be assigned for assessment to a registered practitioner, for example occupational therapist, physiotherapist or social worker, and may include the following situations:

- Where there are unpredictable needs due to neurological, cognitive, emotional or communication problems.
- Where there is an unstable, inconsistent or non-existent social support network.
- Where there is a range of Occupational Performance Issues (OPIs), which together present a complex pathway.
- Where a care package is needed, jointly worked with the social worker, possibly domiciliary care risk assessor or district nurses for example.
- Where a complex adaptation of the home environment is needed.
- Where the patient, family/carers require a high level of advice and support and/or moving and handling education.

The key challenges in the reviews that led to this suggested delegation framework were exploring the fundamental roles of occupational therapy support workers and identifying what needed to change locally. Thus, the delegation framework arose as a result of working with qualified occupational therapists. During these reviews, the therapists were asked to review the tasks they complete every day and to determine if and under what circumstances they could be allocated to another worker. In order to enable such a delegation framework to work in practice, the level of communication between occupational therapists and their support workers needs to be high and open.

The delegation framework was developed due to the need in the current health and social care climate for all levels of staff to be supported to confidently understand and articulate the differences and value in the distinct roles of occupational therapists compared with support workers. In Gloucestershire, the CMOP was useful in underpinning the need to be explicit in differentiating these worker roles within occupational therapy practice. Consequently, a different training programme in the concepts of the model and their role within its use was subsequently created for support staff.

## Facilitation of more seamless care

The model enables the client to identify areas of importance in terms of occupational performance, including self-care, productivity and leisure. In an acute environment, when faced with an unexpected health event, such as a stroke, the client may have a range of short- and long-term OPIs to aim for. Some OPIs may be achievable, with appropriate assessment and advice, during the initial stages of adjustment to disability, such as self-care. Some OPIs may take longer to achieve and need the support of external agencies to maximise return of function and occupational performance, such as leisure.

Collaborative working and flexibility of services is essential to ensure adequate transfer of duty of care across the care pathway. Intervention should be evaluated regularly, and if transfer of care is required, the therapist should be clear that the client needs and any residual risk is handed over to a worker, competent to manage the ongoing issues. Clarity should be given at handover on the outcome of the intervention and residual risk and OPIs.

The client should have consented to a handover of care and be adequately prepared for discharge. The therapist should consider the factors that may trigger re-referral or re-admission to an acute environment and how these have been managed. Therapists should be encouraged to reflect on the learning points from each case and work collaboratively with others to manage barriers to effective care pathways. Working in such a way will ensure all occupational areas are considered, even when the workplace location can appear concerned with limiting the occupational therapist to concentrating on only one occupational performance area such as self-care.

## Conclusion

The challenges of integrating theory into occupational therapy practice were a journey for NHS Gloucestershire over 6 years. Initially, there was a reluctance to challenge current practice in order to evidence client-centred and outcome-focused intervention. Having the right framework in place, to support all levels of staff in managing this change, including consultation, training and a steering group, facilitated the success of implementation. It is anticipated that this success will continue to be sustained.

## References

Awang, D. (2002) Older people and participation within Disabled Facilities Grants processes. *British Journal of Occupational Therapy* 65(6), 261–268.

Bachman, J.P. and Malloch, K.M. (1998) Developing a common nursing practice model. *Nursing Management* 29(1), 1–4.

Beagan, B. and Kumas-Tan, Z. (2005) Witnessing spirituality in practice. *British Journal of Occupational Therapy* 68(1), 17–25.

Buchanan-Barker, P. (2004) The Tidal Model: uncommon sense. *Mental Health Nursing* 24(3), 6–11.

Clarke, C. (2003) Clinical application of the Canadian Model of Occupational Performance in a Forensic Rehabilitation Hostel. *British Journal of Occupational Therapy* 66(4), 171–174.

CSP, RCSLT, BDA and RCN (2006) *Supervision, accountability and delegation of activities to support workers. A guide for registered practitioners and support workers.*

Deegan, C., Watson, A., Nestor, G., Conlon, C. and Connaughton, F. (2005) Managing change initiatives in clinical areas. *Nursing Management* 12(4), 24–33.

Department of Health (2001) *National Service Framework for Older People.* Standard Two: Person Centred Care.

Department of Health (2004) *The NHS Knowledge and Skills Framework (NHS KSF) and the Development Review Process.* Leeds: Department of Health.

Devine, M. and Hirsh, W. (1998) *Mergers & Acquisitions: Getting the People Bit Right.* West Sussex: Roffey Park Management Institute.

Egan, M. and Swedersky J. (2003) Spirituality as experienced by occupational therapists in practice. *American Journal of Occupational Therapy* 57(5), 525–533.

Feaver, S. and Creek, J. (1993) Models for practice in occupational therapy: part 2, what use are they? *The British Journal of Occupational Therapy* 56(2), 59–62.

Hannigan, B. (2004) The ebb and flow of the Tidal Model. *Mental Health Nursing* 24(5), 23.

Health Professions Council (HPC) (2007) *Standards of Proficiency: Occupational Therapists.* London: Health Professions Council.

Hoyland, M. and Mayers, C. (2005) Is meeting spiritual need within the occupational therapy domain? *British Journal of Occupational Therapy* 68(4), 177–180.

Hurst, H. (2003) *Fit for the Future. Strategy Document. Continuing Professional Development for Occupational Therapists.* Unpublished Document commissioned by West Gloucestershire PCT and Gloucestershire Social Services.

Jeris, L., Johnson, J.R. and Anthony, C.C. (2002) HRD involvement in merger and acquisitions decisions and strategy developments: four organisational portraits. *International Journal of Training and Development* 6, 2–12.

Mortenson, W.B. and Dyck, I. (2006) Power and client-centred practice: an insider exploration of occupational therapists' experiences. *The Canadian Journal of Occupational Therapy* 73(5), 261–272.

Mountain, G. (2000). *Occupational Therapy in Social Services Departments: A Review of the Literature.* Centre for Evidence-Based Social Services, Exeter, London: College of Occupational Therapists.

Mullins, L.J. (2005) *Management and Organisational Behaviour,* 7th edn. London: Pearson Education Limited.

Nocon, A. and Pleace, N. (1998) The housing needs of disabled people. *Health and Social Care in the Community* 6(5), 361–369.

Sumsion, T. and Smyth, G. (2000). Barriers to client-centredness and their resolution. *Canadian Journal of Occupational Therapy* 67(1), 15–21.

Taylor, E., Mitchell, J.E., Kenan, S. and Tacker, R. (2000) Attitudes of occupational therapists toward spirituality in practice. *American Journal of Occupational Therapy* 54(4), 421–426.

Thompson, N. (2002) Social work with adults. In: *Social Work: Themes, Issues and Critical Debates,* eds R. Adams, L. Dominelli and D. Payne, 2nd edn, pp. 287–299. Hampshire: Palgrave.

Townsend, E., Stanton, S., Law, M., Polatjko, H., Baptiste, S., Thompson-Franson, T., Kramer, C., Sedlove, F., Brintnell, S. and Campanile, L. (2002) *Enabling Occupation: An Occupational Therapy Perspective.* Ottawa, ON: CAOT, ACE.

Walker, P.J. (2008) *Factors Affecting the Use of the Canadian Model of Occupational Performance by Occupational Therapists Employed by Gloucestershire Primary Care Trust.* Unpublished MSc thesis, University of Plymouth.

Warren, A. (2002) An evaluation of the Canadian Model of Occupational Performance and the Canadian Occupational Performance Measure in Mental Health Practice. *British Journal of Occupational Therapy* 65(11), 515–521.

Wilcock, A.A. and Townsend, E.A. (2009). Occupational justice. In: *Willard and Spackman's Occupational Therapy,* eds E. Crepeau, E. Cohn and B. Schell, 11th edn, pp. 192–215. Philadelphia: Lippincott, Williams and Wilkins.

Wilkins, S., Pollock, N., Rochon, S. and Law, M. (2001). Implementing client-centred practice: why is it so difficult to do? *Canadian Journal of Occupational Therapy* 68(2), 70–79.

# Chapter 10

# Developing occupational therapy theory in Poland

*Ania Pietrzak and Magdalena Loska*

---

**Key points**

- Occupational therapy in Poland is striving to base itself in theory
- In practice occupational therapy is often focussed on craft activities
- Polish occupational therapy would benefit from closer links with the wider occupational therapy community

---

## Introduction

This chapter discusses the emergence of occupational therapy in Poland and the growth and development in the use of theory in this process. We will explore the historical development, how occupational therapy is defined in Poland and the current parameters of our practice and educational systems. We will also describe how we have attempted to introduce occupational therapy theory from around the world into our practice and the challenges we have faced. Finally, we present our suggestions for change that we hope will be a start for developing our rehabilitation systems and encouraging cooperation with other countries that have more experience and advanced practice in occupational therapy.

## Development of rehabilitation and occupational therapy in Poland

The beginnings of occupational therapy in Poland started in the nineteenth century where crafts were used to fill free time in physical rehabilitation and psychiatric programmes. Changes to this approach were made following World War II and can be attributed to pioneering work by Aleksander Hulek, Wiktor Dega and Marian Weiss who developed the Polish rehabilitation system. The creator of the Polish

---

*Using Occupational Therapy Theory in Practice*, First Edition. Edited by Gail Boniface and Alison Seymour.
© 2012 Blackwell Publishing Ltd. Published 2012 by Blackwell Publishing Ltd.

Rehabilitation School, Witkor Dega, described medical rehabilitation as a process where the goals were to improve the body despite disability, ensure dignity of the individual and work towards maintaining a useful and satisfactory life. The ethos in the school was that medicine should see the whole person as a member of the community and he recognised that rehabilitation was a combination of both social and medical processes (Dega 1964).

In 1970, Professor Dega introduced the idea of occupational therapy as a necessary part of the Polish Model of Rehabilitation that was recognised by the World Health Organisation. Occupational therapy was seen as one of four basic rehabilitation forms alongside kinesiotherapy, physiotherapy and orthopaedic supply. He specified two basic aims of occupational therapy:

1. Therapeutic/functional treatment.
2. Vocational rehabilitation that enables the employment of disabled people through education, adaptation and finding suitable employment.

The work of Professor Dega was continued by Kazimiera Milanowska who further emphasised the occupational therapy role within the rehabilitation process. She developed the Polish definition of occupational therapy:

> Occupational therapy is the specified activities, mental or physical, recommended by a medical doctor, carried out by professionals and experts in a specific area. The aim of occupational therapy is to improve and treat and restore the patient's physical and mental efficiency.
>
> (Milanowska 2003, p. 15)

Professor Dega also states that if medical rehabilitation is not integrated with social and vocational rehabilitation then 'the results cannot be full and absolute' (Dega 1964, p. 35).

Unfortunately for many years following the Second World War, occupational therapy was not integrated into rehabilitation services due to lack of funding available through the Polish health care system that did not provide for these services. This was obviously linked to the closed world imposed by the communist government system. This closed system can be seen as being responsible for a limited development of research and development of occupational therapy theory and practice mainly because it did not enable access to Western scientific developments in medicine and rehabilitation practices. Therefore, there was a lack of professional books and publications and a resultant small demand for occupational therapy specialists. Therefore, the effect was that occupational therapy became limited to the organisation of the patient's leisure and was mainly understood in terms of craft or games provision.

Further changes in the development of occupational therapy came about in 1991. The Polish government passed an act regarding social and vocational rehabilitation for people with disabilities that allowed the creation of specific occupational therapy workshops. These workshops were established primarily for people with learning disabilities who were viewed as not capable of work and who would benefit from occupational therapy where social and vocational rehabilitation would be combined. This led to people with learning disabilities becoming more independent, potentially finding a job and living a more satisfactory and integrated life in the community. These workshops filled a gap in current rehabilitation services and they were viewed as the only route for young people with learning disabilities to learn a new profession and find employment.

## Occupational therapy in Poland today

Occupational therapy is still viewed primarily as being craft activities made by people with learning and physical disabilities and the name 'occupational therapist' is generally not understood by the average Pole who tends to only understand the professions of psychology and physiotherapy. Occupational therapy is seen as concentrated on filling the client's free time between medical interventions and physiotherapy. The value of occupational therapy is questioned by the general public who see its role as only being with people with learning disabilities. But is this the reality of occupational therapy practice in Poland?

Currently Polish occupational therapy aims to accomplish the following:

- Physical and functional rehabilitation (this means improving current skills or substituting new skills).
- Vocational rehabilitation (the purpose is to develop work skills and habits for increasing opportunities to enter the work market).
- Social rehabilitation (integration into the wider community).
- Mental and psychological rehabilitation.

Occupational therapists now work in a wider range of service settings in Poland although it is necessary to say that current Polish legislation does not provide for statutory employment of occupational therapists. Therefore, provision is at individual service setting's discretion and is dependent on their financial position. Examples of where occupational therapists are employed are as follows:

- *Hospitals* (but only in orthopaedic services): Their role is to supplement physiotherapy using different craft forms aimed to develop substitutive skills and engage the patient between medical interventions.
- *Hospices*: Here, the occupational therapist's role is to divert the patient's attention away from pain and the debilitating effects of their illness. The most popular interventions are art therapy, music therapy, relaxation and reading. There are often large numbers of occupational therapy volunteers working in these areas.
- *Residential homes for elderly people*: Due to the large numbers of residents in these settings, if an occupational therapist is employed, their role tends to focus on group interventions such as crafts or social events in the community.
- *Residential homes for people with learning and physical disabilities*: Again the role is similar due to the large numbers of residents where it is very difficult to focus the role on individual assessment and intervention.

- *Occupational therapy workshops*: These are support centres for people with disabilities and the only settings in Poland where there is a statutory obligation to provide different forms of occupational therapy for individual clients. Clients spend a few hours per day at the workshop and are divided into different small workshops adapted for different forms of occupation, for example kitchen workshop, craft rooms, pottery workshops and office workshop. In these 'classes' clients learn different forms of daily living activities that will help them socialise and live a normal, active life. Further legislation in 1992 regarding the occupational therapy workshops stipulated their purpose further as follows:
  - General client improvement
  - Development of everyday life skills
  - Preparation for community living
  - Improvement of psychological condition
  - Development of vocational skills aimed at helping clients find work

Although there is admirable work being achieved in these service settings, one of the biggest challenges for occupational therapy in Poland is the lack of standard practices and regulation for occupational therapy staff. We think that there are several reasons for this situation.

Firstly, there is a lack of a national occupational therapy association. We feel that a national association would have the mission of:

- setting standards to unify the education of Polish occupational therapists in line with European and World Federation standards;
- promoting the acknowledgement of Polish occupational therapy diplomas and develop standards to achieve World Federation of Occupational Therapist accreditation;
- promoting occupational therapy theory and practice to improve professional recognition in the wider medical and rehabilitation community;
- promoting, supporting and financing new research to improve the Polish evidence-based occupational therapy practice;
- promoting information exchange between occupational therapists through a professional journal and national conference; and
- aspiring to cooperate with wider occupational communities who have more professional experience in occupational therapy.

A further reason for the current situation in Poland today is the lack of an integrated and holistic political approach for the provision of services for the individual. For example, there are numerous ministries responsible for providing help for people with disabilities. Unfortunately each ministry tends to have its own regulations that are often conflicting. This makes working cooperatively for the benefit of the individual very difficult.

Poland also has a lack of professional occupational therapists who meet the standards according to the World Federation of Occupational Therapists. Currently, there are two ways that people can become occupational therapists, either through medical schools where there is no teaching of occupational therapy theory, social welfare or psychology or through the pedagogical universities where we do not prepare students from a medical perspective. Clearly for occupational therapy education to develop; integrated, holistic curricula are required in order to meet professional educational standards in keeping with other European and world occupational therapists. Linked to this is the difficulty in securing quality practice education experience, with limited occupational therapists being at a standard to take students on placement. There is currently work being done to improve educational standards and through cooperation with the European Network of Occupational Therapy in Higher Education (ENOTHE), some selected universities and colleges are working more in conjunction with other professionals such as physiotherapists and psychologists in order to improve information exchange and encourage multi-disciplinary working.

At present there is no legal regulation of the occupational therapy profession and anyone can be called or employed as an occupational therapist. Therefore, we have the situation where a 'pottery specialist' who has an elementary education only can be employed in an occupational therapy workshop (with no therapeutic training) in the same position as a professional occupational therapist that has a university diploma. In 2005, 135 people who were employed in occupational therapy workshops had an elementary education only and were specialists in one form of occupation such as cooking or broderie.

There is also no universal process of occupational therapy assessment, intervention and evaluation in Poland. We have tried to introduce occupational therapy models such as the Model of Human Occupation (Kielfhofner 2008) and the Canadian Model of Occupational Performance (Townsend et al 1997, 2002). We have learnt about these models through our Erasmus cooperation between ourselves and the occupational therapy department at Cardiff University, but generally, there is a lack of access to professional literature. In addition, limited knowledge of and use of English by occupational therapists and students means that translated texts would be necessary for wider access. This presents difficulties in terms of translation and copyright and the small numbers of texts required in Poland does not make publication in Polish an attractive proposition for publishers.

Attitudes towards people with disabilities are also a barrier to the development of occupational therapy in Poland. A common prevailing attitude towards disability in Poland is to see people with disabilities as victims of their disabilities and circumstances. Thus, they are often viewed as needing care and not being capable of looking after themselves or managing their own affairs (Bhanushali 2007). Most occupational therapists work with people within an institutional setting and there is little necessity seen as to the relevance and value of working with people in their own communities or with their families. Consequently, occupational therapists do not know the full extent of the family, social situation or environmental impact of the disability and, therefore, do not make holistic assessments or intervention plans. The most common aims in Polish occupational therapy are to improve basic functions, to develop interests and to learn new skills (which may not always be relevant to the individual or necessary for independent living). Of course, these leisure and craft occupations are important too because they help develop the spirit and psychological well-being of the client, they improve self-esteem and develop confidence. They help spend time productively, and doing things to give individual satisfaction and they are carried out in an environment where people know and accept the individual, they are not judged and are seen as an individual human being. But is this the help we want to give our clients? At the end of their time in the workshop, they go home to their communities where they are judged by healthy people as being helpless, sick and unpractical or 'stupid'. This is a conse-quence of a general lack of integration within the community as part of an individual therapeutic programme. Even when community trips are organised from the institution, it is always in a group and is not carried out in a 'natural' way. Individuals do not learn independence and self-sufficiency and, therefore, in our opinion clients are stigmatised and marked out as 'disabled'. This attitude then passes on to the client who thinks he cannot do things for himself or live more independently.

## How occupational therapy could improve in Poland through the use of theory

There are many people in Poland who are dedicated to improving occupational therapy education and practice. Unfortunately, these are the people who work every day with people with disabilities but have no power in making decisions or instigating wider political, educational or societal change. As a group of occupational therapists and university staff we engage in discussion about aspects of occupational therapy we could improve:

- How can we make occupational therapy services more efficient?
- How can different institutions collaborate to create a common assessment tool?
- How can occupational therapists do health prevention work?
- How can we monitor and evaluate occupational therapists' activity and work?
- How can we improve cooperation between different specialists and professionals who work with people with disabilities, that is nurses, doctors, physiotherapists, social workers and others?
- How can we improve the cooperation between occupational therapists, the client and the family?
- How can we work in the client's community and how do we regulate this?

In our opinion, the greatest problem we face is the lack of standardised methods of assessment and evaluation of occupational therapy without which we cannot develop adequate therapy or rehabilitation programmes. Due to the political and professional difficulties we have encountered in attempting to translate and utilise international occupational therapy theoretical materials, we have decided to create a new, specific Polish system with our own assessments and instructions. This tool is now being tried out in the occupational therapy workshops.

In the meantime, we would like to improve our connections with other occupational therapists within Poland and in Europe and work together in order to achieve the following:

- We would like to set up some model areas of practice in Poland, where occupational therapists and students can observe and learn how to work with different client groups such as paediatrics and elderly people. These centres would use and develop international tools of assessment and evaluation and work with international staff who are more experienced in order to educate and disseminate good practice.
- We would like to organise and host courses for Polish occupational therapists that are facilitated by international staff. These would be theoretical courses to underpin the practice of occupational therapists in Poland. We think some form of course should be obligatory for every practicing occupational therapist in order to promote continuing professional development.
- We also think there should be greater opportunities for further training for staff involved with occupational therapy education in all universities and institutions in Poland. Currently ENOTHE is working with selected universities and schools and we would welcome widening of this cooperation.
- We would like to organise a conference in Poland that would be open to occupational therapists and educators from Poland and the international community. We would also invite ministers from the government in order to debate issues regarding occupational therapy, rehabilitation and the future development of services for people with disabilities. Financial support through sponsorship would be necessary to organise this event.
- We would also like to pursue how to get international occupational therapy literature in translated form for use in Poland. So far it has been difficult to obtain any information in order to move this forward. This would vastly improve our theory base and practice.

## Conclusion

We have many challenges ahead in order to improve the theoretic understanding and practice of occupational therapy in Poland and to work towards professionalisation and regulation of the profession. This chapter has given us the opportunity to discuss occupational therapy practice in Poland and voice our vision for the future. We hope this begins a new cooperation within the international community of occupational therapists in order to improve services and therapeutic provision for people with disabilities.

## References

Bhanushali, K. (2007) http://wecando.wordpress.com/2007/10/22/disability-movement-from-charity-to-empowerment-by-kishor-bhanushali/ (accessed 8 April 2011).
Dega, W. (1964) *Ortopedia i rehabilitacja*, 1st edn. Warsaw: PZWL.

Kielhofner, G. (2008) *A Model of Human Occupation: Theory and Practice*, 4th edn. Baltimore: Lippincott, Williams and Wilkins.

Milanowska, K. (2003) Materiały konferencyjne z II Ogólnopolskiej Konferencji terapeutów zajęciowych. *Rola i Miejsce terapii zajęciowej w systemie rehabilitacji*, Konin, 2003.

Townsend, E., Stanton, S., Law, M., Polatajko, H., Baptiste, S., Thompson-Franson, T., Kramer, C., Swedlove, F., Brintnell, S. and Campanile, L. (1997) *Enabling Occupation: An Occupational Therapy Perspective*. Ottawa, ON: CAOT ACE.

Townsend, E., Stanton, S., Law, M., Polatajko, H., Baptiste, S., Thompson-Franson, T., Kramer, C., Swedlove, F., Brintnell, S. and Campanile, L. (2002) *Enabling Occupation: An Occupational Therapy Perspective*, 2nd edn. Ottawa, ON: CAOT ACE.

# Chapter 11

# Using occupational therapy theory in Croatia

*Andreja Bartolac*

---

**Key points**

- Terms used in occupational therapy are not necessarily transferable to different countries and cultures
- The history of occupational therapy development in Croatia is bound up with theory and practice
- Theory is important to the development of occupational therapy in Croatia
- Partnerships with other countries assist theory's growth and use

---

## Introduction

The creation and development of the theoretical base and the understanding of occupational therapy in Croatia, together with the development of practice, cannot be explained without an insight into the historical aspects that played a key role in that process. One should bear in mind that Croatia is a small country in the south of Europe and that there are only approximately 250 occupational therapists employed in the health sector. Until very recently, our profession was not legally regulated. This non-regulation of the profession tended to mean that many times jobs for occupational therapists were (and sometimes still are) assigned to experts who were actually not occupational therapy experts, but who came from other professions. Such a situation could often lead to a dilution or even to therapists ignoring the theory of the profession and its associated actions. This situation may not just have been the result of there being only a small occupational therapy population in Croatia, but also a consequence of those therapists' difficulty in clearly arguing and articulating their professional theory and justifying their position in the Croatian health care system. Thus, creating a detrimental effect on the results, they strive for working with a client. This articulation difficulty is often the result of poor knowledge of the theoretical foundations and philosophy of the profession. Consequently, it was not infrequent to have occupational therapists described as *those who are doing something with a client*, where the *something* could be done

---

*Using Occupational Therapy Theory in Practice*, First Edition. Edited by Gail Boniface and Alison Seymour.
© 2012 Blackwell Publishing Ltd. Published 2012 by Blackwell Publishing Ltd.

by some other professional. For example, one could hear descriptions of occupational therapists such as: *they play with children* (as caretakers), *they improve motor skills* (as physical therapists), or *they attract the attention of their clients away from their illness* and *plan their leisure time* (as entertainers). Unfortunately, such lack of understanding of the profession was present not only on the part of other professions but also in clients, and all too often occupational therapists themselves. Reasons for the tacit acceptance of this status quo can be found at various levels: in the educational, medical, social and political systems and in personal motivation and professional self-confidence. At the time when occupational therapists were still seeking their professional identity, the need for occupational therapy services continued to exist and had to be met in one way or another. Therefore, it was other professions, such as social workers, nurses, rehabilitators and many others, that provided the services. However, they tended to cover only certain segments and needs, without having insight into the overall occupational output. Thus, a fragmented approach to occupational therapy was in existence and is, unfortunately, still prevalent in some places even today.

## History of the creation and development of occupational therapy in Croatia

The history of the creation and development of occupational therapy in the world over the past century (Turner et al 2002; Crepeau et al 2003; Creek and Lougher 2008) seems mirrored in the development of the profession in Croatia. Although Croatia could hardly be compared with the United States or the developed countries of the European Union in terms of its resources, it was observed quite early that the inclusion of this activity would yield a health benefit at various levels in the health care system.

In 1915, the physician Bozidar Spisic founded the *Orthopaedic Hospital and Disability School* in Zagreb, thus establishing one of the first institutes in the world to use an early form of occupational therapy. An illustrative example of his philosophical principles can be noted in his emphasis of what he called *work therapy* in rehabilitation; namely, he was convinced that inactivity is very harmful to the whole body and especially to one's mental health. In his words, they were achieving great results by treatment through work, since the patient was beginning to move his joints in a way that was already familiar to him and performing movements that he was used to (Spisic 1917). The patient was working and seeing results in the form of a final product, without even noticing treatment being used.

Like in the United States and other European countries, the ultimate goal of rehabilitation in Croatia at that time was to train disabled World War I veterans to become productive and to have them return to their homes as useful members of the community, that is, reintegration into normal life. Work, mostly some kind of handcraft, was viewed as a healing medium, and training for work was a desirable outcome of rehabilitation. Therefore, it is unsurprising that the treatment method was called *work therapy*. Productivity was prime; therefore, work therapy focused precisely on that field. Such an approach was prevalent for a long time.

In the early 1920s, occupational therapy could also be found in the field of mental health. It was an institutional form of caring for persons, and occupational therapy's focus was on work in its productive and economically self-sustainable form. Work was regarded not only as useful for the functioning of the institution but also as a form of therapy. As stated on the official website of the Jankomir Psychiatric Hospital in 1923, the *colony Jankomir* was founded (Jankomir Psychiatric Hospital 2001). According to the website, occupational therapy was regarded as the only treatment for mental health conditions, but it also had an economic function wherein it provided the means through which food was created to meet patients' needs.

After the introduction of psychopharmaceuticals for people with mental health difficulties, the term *occupation therapy* was introduced. It included a number of activities that were used to fill in the time patients had at their disposal between therapies. The term *occupation* included creative or productive activities the purpose of which was to *occupy* the attention of a client, that is, draw the client's attention away from problems that had led to his or her institutionalisation. Weaving, knitting, wood or metal processing, gardening and manufacturing various products, and later also some artistic media such as clay, cast and painting, were particularly common ways of passing the time in mental health institutions, and also in institutions for children with psychomotor difficulties. Attention was rarely paid to personal preferences and the interests of clients; instead, clients did what was offered to them. Unfortunately, such a rudimentary perception of occupation still exists in certain mental health institutions and it is difficult to eradicate. It suggests that the term *occupation* is still interpreted as it was in its beginnings and that it is not connected with the purposeful activities of everyday life (especially self-care), as it is in other countries. In other words, work and occupation are strictly separated. Translated into the contemporary language of occupational therapy, work refers to productivity, occupation refers to leisure time and self-care is described as a completely special and separate category.

## Issues with the terminology, and a question: what is occupation?

In Croatia, the official name of the profession is *radna terapija* (literally: *work therapy*). However, in certain institutions, various names can still be seen, such as *occupation therapy* or *work-occupation therapy* or *work-productive activities*. The name *work therapy* was probably embraced because of the historically first and basic expected outcome of therapy, which was the ability to work (productivity). Therefore, a more correct equivalent for the name of the profession would be *ergotherapy* (from Greek, *ergon* meaning work). The terms *work*, *activity* and *occupation* in the Croatian language are not synonyms, although they are sometimes used as such. Considering that work primarily relates to the field of productivity (e.g. various types of jobs, housekeeping, studying), it does not seem comprehensive enough to cover all areas in which an occupational therapist works. However, the question *What are you doing?* (literal translation from Croatian would be: *What are you working?*) can be answered in several ways: *I'm repairing a computer, I'm making lunch or I'm singing.*

*Activity* is the most frequently used term having both a general meaning and an applied individual meaning. Occupational therapists in Croatia mostly use it to refer to a wide spectrum of everyday activities that we do while we are awake, so it is most frequently used as a synonym of, and in place of, the term *occupation.*

Defining the term *occupation* presents many difficulties, even controversies. The first association is *to occupy*, that is, to take enemy territory by force. In a state where memories of the War for Independence in the 1990s are still fresh, that meaning has particularly unpleasant historical and social connotations.

The next association is *to occupy oneself* or to become captivated by an activity. This association comes closer to the term occupation as we understand it within the profession, but the explanation is still not sufficiently precise. The term *occupation* in the Croatian language is not a term that would be automatically associated with occupational therapy in everyday speech, and the absence of fluency in using the term results in the unwillingness of even occupational therapists themselves to use it.

Considering that most of the literature in the field of occupational therapy theory is in English, the need to re-elaborate on the meaning of the term *occupation* in occupational therapy when making a translation from the English language resurfaces all the time. It would be extremely practical, as stated by Hagedorn in 1997, if we could use the term occupation as convenient shorthand for describing overall human activity, but in Croatia such automatic understanding is not present. Therefore, the situation where the central term in the philosophy of the profession is not fully embraced creates certain difficulties in both communication and justification of occupational therapy, particularly to other members of the team, and also to users of occupational therapy services, the competent institutions/ministries, employers and sometimes, unfortunately, occupational therapists themselves.

## Development of occupational therapy theory through the perspective of education

Immediately after World War II, emphasis in Croatia returned to the professional rehabilitation of war veterans. Consequently, the School for Physical Medicine and X-ray Imaging was founded in Zagreb in 1947 in which, along with physiotherapists and medical X-ray technicians, occupational therapists began to be officially trained. Although only at the level of 4-year secondary school education, the said school could be regarded as the beginning of formal education for occupational therapists. Still, due to a lack of relevant theory of the profession and a development strategy, over the following 50 years of the past century, development of the profession stagnated.

At the time when Fidler and Fidler (1963) were in the process of defining the theoretical basis of occupational therapy via their discussion of the meaning of and purposeful nature of activity, the use of purposeful activity as a basis for therapy was completely neglected in Croatia, as the focus was on physical rehabilitation. In 1963, the Assembly of the City of Zagreb founded the School Centre for Professional Education of Health Technicians, and the curriculum for occupational therapists was supplemented with medical and professional subjects, with special emphasis on clinical practice (Lovrić 1967). However, little attention was paid to the development of the professional philosophy that would have offered a recognisable identity. Consequently, the education provided in the school resembled more the education of physiotherapists, as it focused on the medical model of education and practice. The health system supported the rehabilitation approach, because it was dominant in all structures and it was strictly separated from the social approach, while the occupational models, within the contemporary meaning of the word, were unknown.

This was particularly visible following the introduction of higher education for oc-cupational therapists in 1986, at the School for Health Studies, which was at the time an operating unit of the Faculty of Medicine at the University of Zagreb. The 2-year study became part of the physiotherapy study, so after graduation, occupational thera-pists acquired the polysemic title 'physiotherapist occupational therapy department'. It made the ambiguity connected with the identity of the profession even greater, because at the end of their studies, students no longer knew whether they were occupational therapists or physiotherapists. It is clear that the situation where occupational therapy did not have an identity of its own, which would clearly differentiate the two pro-fessions, did not suit physiotherapists either. Education of occupational therapists at the time focused on two fields in particular: medical subjects and neuro-rehabilitation, which were taught in line with the syllabus of physiotherapy, and creative activities, which were regarded as a special occupational therapy field. At the time, occupational therapists were taught that the only difference between physiotherapy and occupational therapy was that occupational therapists viewed man holistically and used creativity as a therapeutic medium in their work. The term *holistic* was often used as an argument to identify the profession, and it was explained as abilities (psychosocial and physical) that the occupational therapist acknowledged in their clients.

Focus on abilities and not on occupation at the time did not serve to single out occupational therapy as a profession that provided unique services to a potential client (physical and motor skills are also the subject of interest to physiotherapists, as are psychological and social abilities to psychologists and social workers, sensory skills to rehabilitators and speech is the focus of interest to speech therapists). Soon it became evident that building the theory of the profession solely on various abilities and creative media was not something reserved only for occupational therapy. The question that was becoming more and more topical was: What differentiates the profession of occupational therapy from other professions and what is unique only to occupational therapy in the market of health services?

## External influences on the development of theory of occupational therapy

The turning point in terms of the content of education and changes to the philosophy of occupational therapy in line with the trends prevailing in the professional world were particularly the result of three events: the Croatian–Canadian project of community-based rehabilitation (CBR), connections with the European Network of Occupational Therapy in Higher Education (ENOTHE) and with occupational therapists from Wales.

In parallel with the study of occupational therapy becoming independent of physiotherapy study (in 1997), a great push to the formulation of philosophy of the profession came in 1996 during the 5-year Croatian–Canadian project entitled *Development of Community Based Rehabilitation in the Republic of Croatia* (CBR). The project focused on visibility of rehabilitation as a comprehensive and continued process, combining psychosocial assistance and professional rehabilitation, with the programme of medical rehabilitation (Bobinac-Georgievski 1988). For the first time, a small group of three occupational therapists formed part of the project team. It was the beginning of the process of reformulating the foundations on which the profession is based, so *activity* found itself at the centre of occupational therapy intervention under the influence of the Canadian Model of Occupational Performance (Townsend et al 1997). The focus was finally not solely on the resolution of symptoms or *occupying* in the sense of drawing attention away from an illness.

Encouraged by the Canadian influence, the Canadian Model of Occupational Performance (Townsend et al 2002) was used for the first time in Croatia, and emphasis was placed on the client's personal preference for daily activities and on the outcome, which emphasised participation in the activity, return and active participation in the community, not only on functional restitution. At the time, it was a revolutionary idea for occupational therapists involved in the project, which provided a completely new insight into the profession, and also professional self-confidence. One occupational therapist involved in the project stated:

> For me personally, it was Renaissance. I found out many things about the profession, both theoretical and practical. Two years of formal education did not give me that. Community Based Rehabilitation (CBR) Project offered to me for the first time professional literature on occupational therapy, its field of work (self-care, productivity, and leisure time), activity as a concept, activity analysis, occupational components, contextual factors and other theoretical aspects. I can honestly say that this experience provided me with a wider perspective of how the system functions and with a vision of what it should be; it helped me with the pinpointing of problems and analytical thinking. Actually, the CBR in a way determined my professional identity.
>
> (Personal communication)

In addition, during the project, the Canadian Occupational Performance Measure (Law et al 1998) was translated for the first time, which made it the first assessment of difficulties in the performance of the activities of daily living used in Croatia based on a true occupational therapy model. The CBR project definitely had a positive impact on the introduction of theoretical knowledge to occupational therapy practice, but it took some time for the theoretical concepts to be studied systematically at the level of formal and informal education.

At around the same time, contact with the ENOTHE was established, which had a great impact on the development of the curriculum, and also on raising the awareness of philosophy of the profession. At the very first meeting in Prague (in 1998), and particularly over the following years, it became evident that the Croatian curriculum and its content needed reform, so that the profession of occupational therapy might be identified through an occupation-based programme and competences and thus enabling it to step out of the dominant medical and physiotherapeutic framework. During the intensive period of cooperation with ENOTHE, together with an upgraded 3-year course in occupational therapy (in 1999), changes to the curriculum were slowly carried out. The improvement was primarily at the content level, because the structure of the studies was not flexible in view of the dependence on the approval of the Ministry of Science and Education. Thus, introduction of new occupational therapy theory and philosophy occurred only because of the enlightenment of several teachers.

In 2002, a workshop entitled *The Theory and Philosophy of Occupational Therapy and the Organisation of Fieldwork Practice* was organised for all teachers of occupational therapy subjects. The idea was realised in cooperation with university lecturers at the then University of Wales College of Medicine, Cardiff. The 3-day workshop in Zagreb was attended by 20 teachers and practitioners, where not all of them were occupational therapists, but they did participate in the teaching process. The purpose of the workshop was to improve understanding of the concept and the use of occupation by occupational therapists, along with presenting the basis of occupational therapy theory models and practical approaches in order to identify the relevance of professional theory in practice and education of occupational therapy. Special attention was paid to the clarification of terms used in occupational therapy theory, such as *model, approach, frame of reference* and connectedness with practice. The workshop was purposely organised for teachers in order to help them evaluate their professional role to date and to gain a clearer vision of their future work, as well as to motivate them to share their knowledge with students. The workshop also targeted other experts in the team to sensitise them to the philosophy of occupational therapy through a clarification and demonstration of occupation as a means of therapy and the contribution that occupational therapists can make to an inter- or trans-disciplinary team. At the personal level, the goal was to present occupation as an integral part of the life of any individual, that is, to recognise everyday occupations as an important factor in well-being and health of an individual.

Considering that most participants in the workshop were introduced to the model concept in occupational therapy for the first time (despite some earlier involvement with the Canadian model), we might mark 2002 as the year when occupational therapy theory models were formally presented in Croatia. Still, many therapists showed resistance to new knowledge, and enthusiasm to apply new knowledge in practice was not long lasting. After returning to their workplace, many retained their old pattern of professional thinking and the symptom-oriented approach. Nonetheless, it seems that the results of the workshop had longer lasting consequences on the future generations of students, as the systematic study of occupational therapy models formally began in 2005 following the revision of the curriculum under the influence of the Bologna process. The course *Occupational Therapy Theory and Practice* was introduced for the first time, the purpose of which was to systematically study the occupational therapy theory and make the connection to practice. The syllabus is ambitious in its coverage

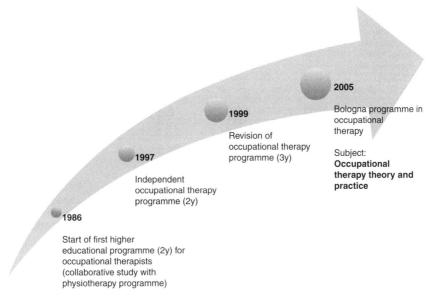

**Figure 11.1**   Development of occupational therapy programme in higher education in Croatia.

of theory of the profession, and at times, it seems that students can find it difficult to understand and apply theory in practice. For example, they can still be confused when they have to select an appropriate occupational therapy model for a particular client. However, one has to bear in mind that only three generations of graduates have participated in the course so far. Thus, students rarely have the opportunity to experience the use of a model in practice. Therefore, they tend to find it easier to embrace the current approach and principle of work that they encounter in the fieldwork than to critically consider the most appropriate selection for the client. Such infrequent use of models might be one of the reasons for therapists' insufficient understanding of theory and for their poor incorporation and use of the appropriate occupational therapy theory as a means of justifying practice, and professional reasoning (Figure 11.1).

The need for teachers to offer a clear and methodologically acceptable clarification of the occupational therapy theory is still present. It is particularly challenging, and also absolutely important to connect the study of the theory of occupational therapy with the other aspects of the curriculum students study, so that they might apply the theory in the various fields of work of an occupational therapist, and not only to associate it with a single course.

## The creation and the role of the Croatian Association of Occupational Therapists

Along with education, one of the most important influences on the development of theory is connected with the activation of occupational therapists in their professional

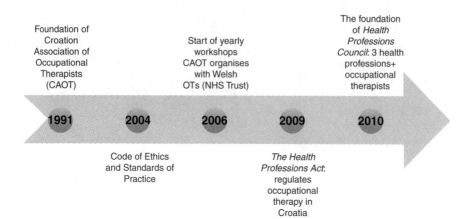

**Figure 11.2** Occupational therapy development and the role of the Croatian Association of Occupational Therapists.

organisation. In the early 1990s, the Croatian Association of Occupational Therapists was formed. It became active only at the beginning of the twenty-first century due to the engagement of several individuals in the management board. As a follow-up to the cooperation with occupational therapists from the University of Wales College of Medicine in Cardiff, strong links were established with occupational therapists in Llandough Hospital in Cardiff. For the last 5 years, the Association has organised annual workshops with occupational therapists from Great Britain. This has resulted in the now almost traditional and ongoing cooperation with Wales. As a consequence, over the past several years there has been much progress. This has primarily been in the strengthening and development of professional self-confidence of individual practitioners, who were presented with an opportunity to learn about professional values and gain new knowledge and skills. Consequently, motivation to stay in the profession and to contribute to the progress of the profession has increased. Dejection that reigned amongst occupational therapists for years, especially young graduates, who were very often forced to work in the field of physiotherapy because of poor prospects of finding a job in the profession, is being overcome (Figure 11.2).

## Conclusion

In preparation of this chapter, a small survey, which identified the use of models by Croatian occupational therapists, was carried out. According to the survey participants, all models identified in this book as occupational therapy professional models were recognised and used to some extent. Therefore, therapists in Croatia must be using some kind of frame of reference for their practice. However, the question is: To what extent are the frameworks based on occupational therapy and how clearly are the therapists following any specific theory?

It seems that there are four types of professional behaviours connected with the use of theory in occupational therapy practice in Croatia:

1. Therapists who use or mostly use the basic postulates of the theory model in practice. However, some of them do not know that it is precisely the said model, that is, they know how to describe the way of their professional thinking and acting, but do not attach a name (or authors) to their applied theory.
2. Therapists who eclectically use several theories, depending on the client and complexity of his or her situation, and thus formulate their *personal theory*.
3. Therapists who are more inclined to identify their professional work against the frame of reference of one of the specialised approaches or techniques (such as sensory integration and neurofacilitation therapy) than with a professional model. They might work in line with a theoretical direction within the meaning of planning the final outcome, but they evaluate their success on the basis of the success achieved at the level of technique.
4. Therapists who do not use any of the theory models and whose primary goal is to improve ability (or reduce medical symptoms), without any occupational perspective.

Regardless of the strategy used, occupational therapists in Croatia definitely need a firm background in the form of a theory through which they can justify their professional actions. The situation in which many therapists still find it unclear where and how to use the theory models as the background for practice is potentially harmful for the profession. This is especially the case in a country where, according to unofficial data, the social welfare system employs over 1000 persons in occupational therapy who do not have any basic training in occupational therapy. This astounding number, which is much higher than the number of employed professional occupational therapists, is the basic motive to regulate the situation in practice. The only way of doing it is through a firm and recognisable theoretical background that will clearly differentiate between the competences of occupational therapists and other professions and will be demonstrated through the examples of good practice.

Despite all obstacles to the use of theory, there are currently many additional changes that have contributed to the return of optimism to Croatian occupational therapists. The adoption of the Health professions Act by the Croatian Parliament in 2009 finally regulated the profession of occupational therapy separately after years of uncertainty. Consequently, occupational therapy in Croatia is currently in the best position ever as it has good foundations in a law that supports its theory. The Act, for example, includes overt reference to the paradigm of the profession, thus providing a strong argument for protecting the professional field of work, the name of the profession and the licence for work. Fortunately, finally there are legal mechanisms that can help in the improvement of the current situation, such as the legislative basis and the public authority of the Croatian Council of Health Professionals. In what way this will influence the practice of Croatian occupational therapists is yet to be seen.

Finally, if asked what has had the greatest impact on the development of the profession both at the level of development of theory and at the level of practice, based on our experience, I would suggest the following:

1. Support provided by occupational therapists from states in which occupational therapy is more developed and enjoys better status. In our case, occupational therapists from Wales played an extraordinary role as they offered selfless professional input, not only in terms of knowledge and experience but also through moral support.
2. Support provided by large occupational therapy organisations at key points of the development of the profession such as the World Federation of Occupational Therapists (WFOT), Council of Occupational Therapists for the European Countries (COTEC), ENOTHE. In our experience, recognising the right moment for action is of upmost importance. For years, the Association advocated unsuccessfully that the profession should be regulated, until the time came for Croatian laws to be aligned with *acquis communautaire*. At that point, we became actively involved (with the strong support of the above-named international organisations) in influencing law-makers in support of the Act, and within 2 months' time, we achieved success, which had been unachievable since the emergence of the profession in Croatia (Figure 11.3).
3. Personal effort of individuals. It has proved to be the case that it is individuals with their personal effort at the workplace and in the course of their free time who promote and develop the profession, inspired by their love of the profession and holding to professional enthusiasm. In our situation, there were several individuals who were involved at all levels of the development of the profession: improving the curriculum, developing cooperation with therapists and organisations outside Croatia, lobbying for the profession, drawing up the act and establishing the Council of Health Professionals.

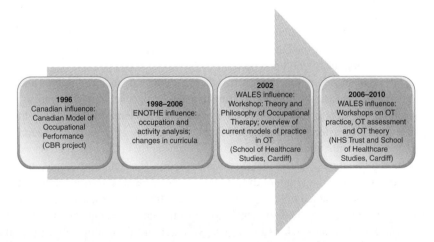

**Figure 11.3**  Influences on using occupational therapy theory in Croatia shown in chronological order.

The process of introducing and applying theory that supports the profession is not an isolated process separated from the history of the profession, the development of education, legislation, demands on the market of services, political and economic influences, lifestyle trends or the way of perceiving one's quality of life. It is also not separate from various external influences, the importance of which was observed only after they stopped being topical, and the cumulative effect of which was observed only after some time and after synchronicity was recognised. Theory should be a well-developed and tested argument that supports practice, but practice (even good practice) can exist even in the cases where theory is not clearly defined by the name and surname of its author, but exists only as a collection of empirical ideas of a professionally motivated expert sensitive to the needs of his or her clients. Still, theory makes it possible to create the identity of a profession and preserve the profession at higher levels, such as social, political and especially inter-professionally; this is unattainable in any other way. If a profession is not substantiated with a clear, proven, recognised and uniform theory, it will be difficult for it to survive. If occupational therapists fail to explain and justify their practice by providing a firm theoretical background, if the students of occupational therapy are not provided with good understanding of the profession on both a theoretical and practical level, if the professional bodies and organisations of occupational therapists fail to protect the identity of the profession by referring to the unique nature of the services that occupational therapy offers within other health and social professions (substantiated by a single occupational therapy theoretical basis), the survival of the profession can be at risk.

## Acknowledgements

Thanks to Gail Boniface, who at the time occupied the position of Senior Lecturer, and Ruth Crowder, who was Lecturer and Fieldwork Leader, at the then University of Wales College of Medicine, Cardiff, for their cooperation in setting up the 2002 workshop in Zagreb entitled *The Theory and Philosophy of Occupational Therapy and the Organisation of Fieldwork Practice*. Thanks also to the exceptional contribution of Helen Hortop, Head of OT Services, Cardiff, and Vale University Health Board and the Artificial Limb and Appliance Services.

## References

Bobinac-Georgievski, A. (ed.) (1988) *Community Based Rehabilitation: Development in the Republic of Croatia*. Prva hrvatsko-kanadska tematska konferencija o projektu Razvoj rehabilitacije u zajednici u RH za pozvane sudionike. Opca bolnica 'Sveti Duh'. 1–2.

Creek, J. and Lougher, L. (eds) (2008) *Occupational Therapy and Mental Health*. Edinburgh: Churchill Livingstone.

Crepeau, E.B., Cohn, E.S. and Schell, B.A. (eds) (2003) *Willard & Spackman's Occupational Therapy*. Philadelphia: Lippnicott, Williams and Wilkins.

Fidler, G. and Fidler, J. (1963) *Occupational Therapy: A Communication Process in Psychiatry.* Toronto: Macmillan.

Hagedorn, R. (1997) *Foundations for Practice in Occupational Therapy.* New York: Churchill Livingstone.

Jankomir Psychiatric Hospital (2001) http://www.mcs.hr/jankomir/povijest.asp?action=povijest (accessed 18 December 2009).

Law, M., Baptiste, S., Carswell, A., McColl, M., Polatajko, H. and Pollock, N. (1998) *Canadian Occupational Performance Measure*, 3rd edn. Ottawa, ON: CAOT ACE.

Lovric, S. (1967) *20-godišnjica Skole za fizikalnu medicinu i röndgen u Zagrebu*; razdoblje: 1947–1967, Zagreb.

Spisic, B. (1917) *Kako pomazemo nasim invalidima? Slike iz nase ortopedijske bolnice iinvalid-skih skola. Dionicarska tiskara* Zagreb, Zagreb.

Townsend, E., Stanton, S., Law, M., Polatjko, H., Baptiste, S., Thompson-Franson, T., Kramer, C., Sedlove, F., Brintnell, S. and Campanile, L. (1997) *Enabling Occupation: An Occupational Therapy Perspective*. Ottawa, ON: CAOT ACE.

Townsend, E., Stanton, S., Law, M., Polatjko, H., Baptiste, S., Thompson-Franson, T., Kramer, C., Sedlove, F., Brintnell, S. and Campanile, L. (2002) *Enabling Occupation: An Occupational Therapy Perspective*, 2nd edn. Ottawa, ON: CAOT ACE.

Turner, A., Foster, M. and Johnson, S.E. (eds) (2002) *Occupational Therapy and Physical Dysfunction: Principles, Skills and Practice*. Edinburgh: Churchill Livingstone.

## Further reading

COTEC, located at http://www.cotec-europe.org/.

ENOTHE, located at http://www.enothe.eu/.

WFOT, located at http://www.wfot.org/.

# Chapter 12

# Personal reflections on understanding and using the Model of Human Occupation in practice

*Sarah Cook*

---

**Key points**

- Using model-based assessments in isolation from the occupational therapy model of practice can create a superficiality to practice
- A model is a toolbox within which to structure thinking and is therefore used as a model *for* not *of* practice
- We should not slavishly just adhere to models but use them in a reflexive way

---

## Introduction

The aim of this chapter is to share some of my experiences and reflections of using the Model of Human Occupation (MOHO) (Kielhofner 2008) within various mental health settings. It will aim to explore the following:

- The drivers for using a model in practice.
- How the model was applied to my practice.
- How the model influenced my theoretical knowledge.
- How the model impacted on the therapeutic relationships formed with service users.
- How the model influenced the problem-solving process and the outcome of therapy.
- How the use of the model impacted on the management of practice and resources.

## What are the drivers for using a model in occupational therapy practice?

In 1994, Mattingly and Fleming found that occupational therapists placed little if any value on the role or relevance of theory to practice. In 1999, the Department of Health called for services to develop an integrated approach to their organisational and

---

*Using Occupational Therapy Theory in Practice*, First Edition. Edited by Gail Boniface and Alison Seymour.
© 2012 Blackwell Publishing Ltd. Published 2012 by Blackwell Publishing Ltd.

professional development (DH 1999). In addition, the British College of Occupational Therapists called for the gap to be bridged between practice and theory (COT 2002). The Health Professions Council (HPC 2007) also requires practitioners to utilise theoretical concepts and standardised assessments and suggests that the use of established theories and models of occupational therapy is a standard of clinical proficiency.

As a student in the mid-1990s, I was encouraged to explore the use of occupational therapy models and approaches. I attended lectures and workshops that stressed the importance of using theory to underpin practice. Various concepts were explored, discussed and related to case examples in an attempt to demonstrate that the theory had been understood. I subsequently encountered the MOHO (Kielhofner 2008) being used in practice in the occupational therapy department where I took up my first post. In that setting, standardised assessments associated with the model were undertaken in an attempt to communicate an understanding of the concepts that made the model unique. The Occupational Self-Assessment (Baron et al 2006), the Role Checklist (Oakley 1981) and the Interest Checklist (Kielhofner and Neville 1983) were the tools primarily used for assessment. Additionally, significant value was placed on the collaborative nature of these as well as their capacity for self-rating. All of these assessments I encountered at that time felt client-focused, because the completion of any of these assessments resulted in a list of the service users' significant roles and interests and a list of goals to work on in therapy. The information gathered was always sufficient to work with. However, due to us using the assessments in isolation from the model, it felt superficial to me as we lacked deeper exploration and analysis of the theory underpinning the assessments.

It was not until I was challenged about my role in a ward round by an enthusiastic consultant some 4.5 years into my career that my process of reflecting on using the model began. It caused me to raise questions for myself, such as *What influenced my thinking in practice? How did I structure the way I worked with service users?* I realised I needed a defined assessment process that would give a broader understanding of occupational performance, something that highlighted more about the person than just identifying what they were engaged in doing. I realised *doing* was an important part of occupational therapy, but I wanted to know more about *why* service users were *doing* chosen occupations, how they were *doing* those occupations and what influenced their abilities to *do* occupations. The first assessment to broaden my understanding of this and the role of an occupational therapist was the Model of Human Occupation Screening Tool (MOHOST) (Parkinson et al 2006) that remains my functional assessment of choice. I recall an occupational therapist in a previous post referring to the MOHOST (Parkinson et al 2006) as an assessment 'grounded in practice'. Thus, I initiated use of this assessment, referring to the manual's extended criteria to aid me in its completion. My motivation to convey clarity of my role to the consultant assisted in my keenness to explore the theory behind the assessment further. I also recall feeling frustrated generally with my lack of understanding of my professional role, often joking with a colleague that someone would 'find me out' and expose my superficial understanding of occupational therapy practice. I was soon reassured of my sound practice but the lack of theoretical structure created a somewhat chaotic and woolly delivery, leaving me unsure of the effectiveness of my work. The next section will consider the journey I underwent to establish a sounder theoretical structure to my way of working.

## How has the model influenced my theoretical knowledge of occupational therapy?

I began using the MOHOST (Parkinson et al 2006) regularly as my main tool for assessment. When a service user is able to engage in an interview-based process I primarily use the Occupational Circumstances Assessment – Interview Rating Scale (OCAIRS) (Forsyth et al 2005) that informs my MOHOST (Parkinson et al 2006) report. This information is supplemented with information extrapolated from observations in the clinical setting and by third party proxy reporting. Thus, I consider the MOHO's assessments as my *toolbox* and choose the appropriate assessment based on what information I need to know, and the best way in which to gather this information. Another assessment I regularly use is the Volitional Questionnaire (De las Heras et al 2003), which is used mainly with the Remotivation Process (De las Heras 2003), which I will return to later in this chapter.

The MOHOST was developed in the United Kingdom by Occupational Therapists in the clinical field (Parkinson et al 2006). It provides an overview of the factors that influence an individual's function in the areas of volition, habituation, performance and environment and looks at how they combine to influence an individual's occupational participation (Parkinson et al 2006). It is designed to be scored from a variety of information sources, for example informal observation, interviewing or reviewing the clinical notes. I use the assessment to consolidate information I have on an individual and structure my report around the six areas that together form a comprehensive summary of the individual's occupational profile. Using this assessment has provided a good overview of the model's concepts and has allowed me to strengthen my understanding of the theory underpinning the model.

I was working in a forensic setting when I first used the MOHOST (Parkinson et al 2006). I worked on a mixed long-term specialist rehabilitation ward where I had the time to get to know service users and develop an in-depth understanding of their world. A significant factor to be considered when working with service users in a forensic setting is the impact of the environment on occupational functioning; both in relation to the restrictions created by the physical environment and the restrictions imposed by the various forensic sections. Prior to the development of the MOHO (Kielhofner 2008), other occupational therapy theories tended to focus on impairment. However, the MOHO (Kielhofner 2008) emphasised that it was not only the characteristics of an individual that were important but also the impact that the environment had on an individual and how that influenced their participation in occupation. This resonated for me, working within the restricted setting of a secure service, I came face to face with the realities of how an environment either supported or restricted a service users' engagement in occupation. Even the most basic self-care tasks were impacted, not only by the obvious effects of lack of motivation but also the impact of risk management strategies on the unit, which meant having to request access to tools required for those activities. For example, requesting shaving foam, deodorant or razors that were locked in secure areas and asking to be let into the locked bathroom to perform the self-care task. The model allowed me to explore these issues in a complex way, teasing out components of a task and the opposing and affording factors, often resulting in observations overlooked by the rest of the clinical team. The discussions that followed were often useful in determining ways in which we could support service users to complete essential self-care tasks safely, with the least security restrictions possible.

When offered a locum post in neuropsychiatry in 2009 I was somewhat apprehensive about my ability to work in that setting. I had no prior experience in that area and felt I had little to offer in the way of clinical expertise. I was encouraged to accept the post and was reassured that my experience of completing Assessments of Motor and Processing Skills (Fisher 1995; Bray et al 2001) and the support I would receive from colleagues would get me through. Creek (2003) suggests that the use of a model can be likened to using a map, in that it guides the therapeutic process by providing a framework within which to work. I was surprised to find the model enabled me to construct a map or a platform for understanding functional ability in that area, allowing me to quickly understand the needs of the service users. I was able to use the assessments with which I was already familiar, the MOHOST (Parkinson et al 2006) and the OCAIRS (Forsyth et al 2005) to provide the clinical team with a profile of a service user's occupational functioning. Over the 6 months, I worked in the area and began to notice trends in the information I had gathered. This helped me to focus my attention on the areas of dysfunction and supported me to collaborate quickly with service users regarding appropriate rehabilitation strategies. In fact I began finding that the model was having an impact on the way in which I was working with service users, something the next section will elaborate on.

## The impact of the model on the therapeutic relationship with a service user

The majority of my career has been spent working with people deemed as *treatment resistant*, a term with which I am very uncomfortable. Of course this refers to the resistance of pharmaceutical intervention, but it often affects the team's perception of the overall improvement that a service user can make. The MOHOST (Parkinson et al 2006) creates a *real picture* of how service users function throughout their lives and provides some meaningful narrative. Often service users would refer to hope or optimism; seemingly positive determinants in assessing an individual's ability to improve and it enabled me to capture these concepts. I wanted to share the flickers of hope observed in my daily interactions; the signs that indicated to me there was some capacity and willingness to change and therefore challenge the perception of treatment resistance. I was often at a loss as to how to capture and describe these concepts of hope and seemingly minimal signs of change. However, I found that the MOHOST (Parkinson et al 2006) encourages consideration of hope and optimism and explores change in detail. It covers service users' capacity to change, explores the supports needed to change and also considers the service user's tolerance level for change. This enabled different conversations with the team and supported me to think about grading interventions to address those difficulties. The assessment also explores values, choice and opportunities that helped me to explore issues related to quality of life, which I was then able to relate to the extremely restrictive forensic setting. In the absence of active rehabilitation, quality of life becomes the essential consideration for this client group.

Assertive Outreach teams work with service users who display difficulties engaging in the therapeutic process. Whilst working as an occupational therapist in that team I often found it a challenge to establish rapport and initiate the formal assessment process. The service users' tolerance for support and intervention was minimal and I needed to explore other avenues for eliciting information. An additional issue for this service user group was the ability to self-report accurately. Often a rosy picture would be painted by the service user through initial enquiry, which was not evidenced in reality. Using the MOHOST (Parkinson et al 2006), allowed consideration of material that reflected the service user's perspective and in addition I was able to record my observations, ensuring both perspectives were captured. It encouraged the exploration of alternatives to interview-based methods that was a novel way of working and challenged my perception of occupational therapy. I had always embraced the idea of *doing* with service users and initially felt lost in my new observer role. I questioned whether assessments could be completed without questions being asked. This is often queried by junior staff and students in my team, but what they and I had neglected to realise was that this form of assessing via service users *doing* or engaging in occupations, allowed information to be collected from a *range* of different sources. Questions could supplement my observations, but I could also use information gathered from a range of everyday interactions to start to build a picture of the service user's world. It allowed me to observe service users informally in everyday activity, without the need to intrude or ask of them, anything out of their usual routine. In a ward setting I could use community meetings, meal times and smoking breaks, and could spend time in the social areas of the ward to complete observations that would inform the assessment process. The expanded criteria of the assessment helped me to organise the observed material into a comprehensive assessment format.

Establishing meaningful therapeutic alliances with service users who have forensic histories or personality vulnerabilities can be challenging (see also Chapter 5). Often abusive or exploitative relationships are all that has been experienced by service users in this setting. Working in this area posed initial difficulties for me, particularly with understanding and empathising with service users whose offences challenged my values and norms, and secondly, engaging in relationships where I was often the target of manipulation and exploitation. I wanted to understand how offending related to occupational performance, how the person's values and beliefs influenced their life patterns and performance and how these were hindered or enhanced by the environment. Service users in this setting often struggled to relate to their clinical team, displaying difficulties with trust, respect and collaborative working. The model enables the therapist to explore these concepts and considers these elements theoretically, enabling focus to be given to these areas of intervention. It also encourages therapists to explore values and experiences that may be unique to an individual and examine their impact on occupational functioning. This exploration was useful in a setting where the inevitable questions are asked about how someone could commit such an offence. It helped question motivations for engaging in a variety of antisocial and criminal occupations. The MOHOST (Parkinson et al 2006) assisted exploration of the gains to be had and the thrill of rule breaking and explored circumstances that may have given rise to offending such as lack of structure, roles, challenges or opportunities. It also helped me to think about how the status attached to the role of an offender serves as a motivator to committing criminal acts and the role that power plays in that scenario. It also helped me to explore the sense of belonging that is felt either by social groups, fellow offenders or gangs and the structure and expectation those relationships afford. Whilst the model prompted me to explore these issues as they are core to its theory, it also supported me to retain my client-centred focus encouraging me to find out all I could about what was important to the individual allowing me to explore and understand rather than judge and punish.

## How the problem-solving process and the outcome of therapy are influenced by the model

I have referred extensively in this chapter to how the model has influenced my assessment process but have spoken little of how it has impacted on the rest of the problem-solving process. In part I think this reflects the weight of information and guidance there is about assessing using the model, but I have found it helpful in guiding and influencing each part of the clinical process. Thomer (1991) provides the reminder that assessments provide little benefit if they do not inform the treatment process and lead to the setting of collaborative goals. The findings of the MOHOST (Parkinson et al 2006) should inform the development of intervention goals, but little guidance is provided in this area. I have found that a common criticism of the model from my occupational therapy colleagues is its focus on assessment rather than intervention. For this reason, I have used other methods for setting goals, for example Goal Attainment Scaling (Kiresuk and Sherman 1968), but have attempted to group the goals under the MOHOST (Parkinson et al 2006) sub-headings.

Developing intervention programmes that challenged and supported service users, involved thinking about the relationship between motivation, habits and roles, the environment and occupational performance. The use of the model alongside my other core occupational therapy skills enabled me to design programmes that targeted specific areas of dysfunction and provided opportunities to build on functional strength. For example, introducing self-evaluation to sessions encouraged reflection and aided the improvement of a service users self-appraisal. In addition, grading challenge into an activity provided a means for increasing frustration tolerance in activity. In the forensic setting, the model supported me to think about providing opportunities for service users to experience success in activities of value to an individual. Service users were supported to engage in non-criminal activity that did not place value on antisocial behaviours but were valuable to the individual's value and belief systems. An example of this was supporting a male service user to complete a referees' course in football. He was able to fulfil a lead role in an activity that supported his need to be in a position of authority but in a role that required him and others to play by the rules.

An area of intervention that has been particularly influenced by the model is the work to address issues with motivation. The model provides a clear format for viewing and understanding volition, and the Remotivation Process (De las Heras et al 2003) provides guidance for understanding motivation stages and outlines intervention to address volitional challenge. The Remotivation Process was designed for service users' with severe volitional problems and was developed in response to a lack of recognised intervention strategies. It is a structured process of intervention developed to improve motivation for occupational engagement. The process requires the therapist to understand and support a service user's experience. It seeks to support a reconnection with the world while gradually increasing a person's sense of personal causation, values and interests. It consists of three phases: (a) exploration, (b) competency and (c) achievement; each of which is made up of stages with specific intervention strategies (De las Heras et al 2003). Thus I found clear occupational resonance in both the assessment and the model in that if the MOHOST (Parkinson et al 2006) highlighted deficits in the area of volition, I was prompted to complete a Volition Questionnaire (De las Heras et al 2003). If in addition specific difficulties in relation to motivation were highlighted, I would consult the Remotivation Process (De las Heras et al 2003). The process allowed me to view service users along a continuum of change and helped me to ascertain their current volitional capacity, providing me with stage specific objectives for intervention. I was able to apply the re-motivation theory to both individual and group interventions within the existing ward programme. I was able to use the theory to clearly articulate to the team the difficulties experienced by the service user and was able to grade the interventions delivered using the guides for each stage from the process. The therapy strategies and client aims outlined in the model and assessment manuals supported me to implement structured and focused interventions that also formed the basis of the group protocols. The theory supported the enhancement of my clinical reasoning for applying specific strategies and provided a ready-made measure of outcome. Although there was a structure to follow, it was flexible enough to accommodate service user needs. As I became more proficient in its use, so my ability to recognise, monitor and record change improved. Using the Remotivation Process (De las Heras et al 2003) in practice significantly enhanced my understanding of the concept of volition in practice and how it could be improved.

Each of the model's standardised assessments have scoring systems that can be used to document and map changes to service users' performance. This has enabled me to use the assessments as an outcome measure to support justification for my input. Clarke et al (2001) suggests that it is a challenge to discover the appropriate tools to measure the quality of our work, but I disagree. I have valued the MOHOST (Parkinson et al 2006) and Volitional Questionnaire (De las Heras et al 2003) assessments as outcome measures and use them regularly to document scores for performances pre- and post-intervention. The MOHOST (Parkinson et al 2006) details a breakdown of occupational concepts and allows simple rating of these allowing swift identification of strengths and areas of dysfunction. Changes in performance can also be promptly identified, demonstrating with ease a measure of outcome for occupational therapy intervention. The clear concepts outlined in the MOHOST (Parkinson et al 2006) report allow the format to be easily understood by other professions, further justifying the effectiveness of occupational therapy interventions. This leads me into the next section on the impact of the model on management related issues.

## How the model impacts on the management of practice and resources

This model has significantly influenced service delivery, planning and management for the departments I have worked in. Completing multiple MOHOST (Parkinson et al 2006) assessments across different settings has assisted me to build a picture of service users functioning, often highlighting performance themes in the areas where I have worked. The themes are sometimes obvious and are reflected in other types of care theories. For example, difficulties establishing relationships is associated with the negative symptoms of schizophrenia. But other examples such as poor tolerance for change associated with service users I worked with in neuropsychiatry and long-term rehabilitation were also evident through the assessment analysis but are less defined in general psychiatric literature. Using the MOHO ensures a substantial amount of information is gathered about the influence of the environment on an individual's functioning. This has been of assistance in discussions within the teams within which I have worked, about options for adaptation or alteration within that environment to support a client's maximum functioning. I have also found that the identification of themes has also assisted with more effective intervention planning and improved targeting of resources.

Overall, using the model has helped me maintain a clear occupational therapy role assisting me in providing effective occupation-focused interventions. My occupational therapy colleagues often speak about role blurring and have reported feeling disillusioned by it. Although I recall experiencing those feelings early in my practice, I now feel, through the continued use of the model, confident with my sense of professional, occupational identity. Generic working is a major threat for disciplines working in community teams. Whilst working in a multi-disciplinary assertive outreach team, a *team approach* was used; a method of working that meant the whole team supported individuals to enable daily care needs to be met. I encountered pressure from colleagues to fully participate in this, which reduced the time I had for core occupational therapy input. At times I encountered criticism for ring-fencing occupation-focused work, but my clear MOHO (Kielhofner 2008) based aims and objectives provided reasoning and justification for my sessions, which were then accepted. Often the prospect of utilising a model in practice will generate discussion about the time constraints involved with learning the theory and using the lengthy assessment formats. This issue is frequently brought up in the training workshops I have facilitated and in supervision sessions with staff. Whilst I recognise this as a factor, the learning of any new information or skill requires time and effort for it to be effective. I have spent time reading the model's manuals and reviewing case studies. I have often specifically done so when considering how I have incorporated the theory into my reporting. Overall, therefore, I have found the benefits of using theory to guide practice for individual occupational therapists' and occupational therapy departments, greatly outweigh the initial study time required to understand the theory of any occupational therapy model of practice.

## Conclusion

Having used the MOHO (Kielhofner 2008) in practice for over 11 years, it has only been in the last 7 years that I can truly say I understand it. Previously my use was limited to referencing the model, using some of the standardised assessments and structuring reports around the sub-systems outlined in the theory. Thankfully, through perseverance, the continued use of the assessments and the experience of using the MOHOST (Parkinson et al 2006) assessment in particular, I fully understand the relevance of the theory to service users and appreciate the clarity it provides in relation to my role as an occupational therapist. I am aware that this chapter has provided limited criticism of the model's use, and this accurately reflects my experience of it. I have found using the model a largely positive experience and have very little to criticise.

The theory has provided me with a confidence in my practice that is often commented on by others. It has provided a clear format for communication with service users, a language with which to articulate service user needs and the MOHOST (Parkinson et al 2006) in particular has provided a framework that is understood by my multi-disciplinary team colleagues.

One of the central features of the model is the extent to which occupational therapy practitioners are encouraged to research and develop it. There is already a wealth of information generated about its effectiveness, and there is the potential to research the need for occupational therapy services by providing evidence of the effectiveness of practice using this model. I hope to be able to continue to contribute to this to evidence and urge occupational therapists to challenge the perception of occupational therapy by others, as a woolly profession. Hopefully then the lack of respect for occupational therapy will cease, paving the way for the recognition it deserves.

# References

Baron, K., Kielhofner, G., Lyengar, A., Goldhammer, V. and Wolenski, J. (2006) *The Occupational Self Assessment (OSA) (version 2.2)*. Chicago: Model of Human Occupation Clearinghouse. Department of Occupational Therapy, College of Applied Health Sciences, University of Illinois at Chicago.

Bray, K., Fisher, A.G. and Duran, L. (2001) The validity of adding new tasks to the assessment of motor process skills. *American Journal of Occupational Therapy 2001, July–August* 55(4), 409–415.

Clarke, C., Sealey-Lapes, C. and Kotsch, L. (2001) *Outcome Measures Information Pack for Occupational Therapy*. London: College of Occupational Therapists.

College of Occupational Therapists (COT) (2002) Position statement on lifelong learning. *British Journal of Occupational Therapy* 65(5), 198–200.

Creek, J. (2003). *Occupational Therapy Defined as a Complex Intervention*. London: College of Occupational Therapists.

De las Heras, C.G., Geist, R., Kielhofner, G. and Li, Y. (2003) *The Volitional Questionnaire (VQ) (version 4.0)*. Chicago: Model of Human Occupation Clearinghouse. Department of Occupational Therapy, College of Applied Health Sciences, University of Illinois at Chicago.

De las Heras, C.G., Llerena, V. and Kielhofner, G. (2003) *The Remotivation Process: Progressive Intervention for Individuals with Severe Volitional Challenges (version 1.0)*. Chicago: Model of Human Occupation Clearinghouse. Department of Occupational Therapy, College of Applied Health Sciences, University of Illinois at Chicago.

Department of Health (DH) (1999) *National Service Frameworks for Mental Health: Modern Standards and Service Models*. London: Department of Health.

Fisher, A.G. (1995) *Assessment of Motor and Process Skills*. Fort Collins, CO: Three Star Press Inc.

Forsyth, K., Deshpande, S., Kielhofner, G., Henriksson, C., Haglund, L., Olson, L., Skinner, S. and Kulkarni, S. (2005) *The Occupational Circumstances Assessment – Interview and Rating Scale (OCAIRS) (version 4.0)*. Chicago: Model of Human Occupation Clearinghouse. Department of Occupational Therapy, College of Applied Health Sciences, University of Illinois at Chicago.

Health Professions Council (HPC) (2007) *Standards of Proficiency: Occupational Therapists*. London: Health Professions Council.

Kielhofner, G. (2008) *A Model of Human Occupation*, 4th edn. Baltimore: Lippincott, Williams and Wilkins.

Kielhofner, G. and Neville, A. (1983) *The Modified Interest Checklist*, Unpublished manuscript, Model of Human Occupation Clearinghouse, Department of Occupational Therapy, University of Illinois at Chicago.

Kiresuk, T. and Sherman, R. (1968) Goal Attainment Scaling: a general measure of evaluating comprehensive mental health programs. *Community Mental Health Journal* 4, 443–453.

Mattingly, C. and Fleming, M. (1994) *Clinical Reasoning: Forms of Inquiry in a Therapeutic Practice*. Philadelphia: F.A. Davis Company.

Oakley, F. (1981) *The Role Checklist*. The Model of Human Occupation Clearinghouse, Department of Occupational Therapy, College of Applied Health Sciences, University of Illinois at Chicago.

Parkinson, S., Forsyth, K. and Kielhofner, G. (2006) *The Model of Human Occupation Screening Tool (MOHOST) Version 2.0*. Chicago: The Model of Human Occupation Clearinghouse.

Department of Occupational Therapy, College of Applied Health Sciences, University of Illinois at Chicago.

Thomer, S. (1991) The essential skills of an occupational therapist. *British Journal of Occupational Therapy* 5(6), 222–223.

## Further reading

Parkinson, S., Forsyth, K. and Kielhofner, G. (2006) *The Model of Human Occupation Screening Tool (MOHOST) Version 2.0.* Chicago: The Model of Human Occupation Clearinghouse. Department of Occupational Therapy, College of Applied Health Sciences, University of Illinois at Chicago.

# Contemporary Discussions on the Use of Theory in Occupational Therapy Practice

# Chapter 13

# Using occupational therapy theory within evidence-based practice

*Carly Reagon*

---

**Key points**

- The evidence base for occupational therapy is wide ranging
- Conceptions of evidence-based practice are influenced by larger philosophical debates about the nature of science
- Occupational therapists can use conceptual models of the profession as a framework for evidence-based practice
- Occupational therapy theory can help to identify and inform the search for and development of evidence within the profession

---

## Introduction

This chapter explores the relationship between evidence-based practice and the use of professional theory by occupational therapists. Whilst it does not offer instruction about how to do evidence-based practice (see the end of the chapter for suggestions for further reading on this subject), it demonstrates the critical role that theory has to play in developing an approach to evidence-based practice that is specific to and compatible with occupational therapy. The chapter starts by describing evidence-based practice and its role in health care today, before moving on to suggest ways in which theory can, and indeed should, inform such evidence-based practice. The first of these is the use of theory to underpin the science of evidence-based practice for occupational therapists; the second is the use of an occupational therapy professional conceptual model within evidence-based practice; the third is the use of theory in seeking the evidence base and the fourth is the relationship between theory and research evidence.

---

*Using Occupational Therapy Theory in Practice*, First Edition. Edited by Gail Boniface and Alison Seymour.
© 2012 Blackwell Publishing Ltd. Published 2012 by Blackwell Publishing Ltd.

# What is evidence-based practice?

Evidence-based practice is an approach to professional practice in which decisions are based upon evidence such as research findings rather than unsubstantiated opinion or tradition. Given the increasing demand for health care worldwide and the increased awareness of ineffective, inefficient or even harmful health care practices, evidence-based practice has become extremely popular over the last 20 years. One of the most cited definitions of evidence-based practice is 'the conscientious, explicit, and judicious use of current best evidence in making decisions about the care of individual patients' (Sackett et al 1996, p. 71). In a later description, the authors added in the phrase 'best research evidence' and its integration with clinical expertise, patient values and individual circumstances (Sackett et al 2000). An alternative definition offered by Reagon et al (2008) presents evidence-based practice in occupational therapy as part of the client-centred process in which evidence from multiple sources is systematically gathered, examined and used to 'illuminate information-rich choices for clients and their therapists' (p. 435).

## What is evidence?

In most of the earlier literature, the term 'evidence' is reserved for research findings, particularly those from robustly designed quantitative studies such as randomised controlled trials. However, qualitative research is increasingly recognised as a useful source of evidence particularly with the emergence of mixed method research (Creswell 2011). Some authors have also argued that professional opinion, client feedback and even intuition are legitimate sources of information that can be used alongside research evidence to inform practice (Greenhalgh 2002; Reagon et al 2008). However, as will be explored later in this chapter, this is an area of continued debate, reflecting different professional backgrounds and conceptions of health care.

## The development of evidence-based practice

Using evidence to inform professional practice is not a new concept and can be traced as far back as the ancient world. However, in plotting its more recent history, it is clear that evidence-based practice developed within the medical profession (as evidence-based medicine) and grew outwards to encapsulate other disciplines. Recent enthusiasm for evidence-based practice has been attributed to various factors including rising consumer interest in effectiveness and quality of health care, high profile cases of medical negligence and malpractice, changing attitudes towards expertise (patients no longer trust *experts* implicitly), the increasing global accessibility of information, new technologies and new knowledge and increased demand for health care (Trinder 2000; Gray 2001). The challenge of providing evidence-based services reverberates across government and professional literature, including literature from within the field of occupational therapy. For example, the Code of Ethics and Professional Conduct

---

**Box 13.1** **Model of evidence-based practice based on Sackett et al (2000)**

Step 1    Ask an answerable clinical question, for example about diagnosis,
          prognosis, prevention or therapy.
Step 2    Find the current best evidence to answer that question. Sackett et al
          (2000) offer various ways of tracking this evidence down and making the
          process manageable.
Step 3    Critically appraise the evidence. This should be carried out in various
          ways including assessing the evidence in terms of validity, impact and
          relevance to practice.
Step 4    Integrate the critical appraisal with therapeutic expertise and
          consideration of the client's unique circumstances. (Inclusion of this step
          confronts criticisms of evidence-based practice that describe it as a highly
          prescriptive or *cook book* approach to practice.)
Step 5    Evaluate the practitioner's performance of Steps 1–4 via reflection and
          identify ways to improve the process.

---

for Occupational Therapists (College of Occupational Therapists 2010) in the United Kingdom stipulates that 'any advice or intervention provided should be based upon the most recent evidence available, best practice, or local/national guidelines and protocols' (p. 17, Section 3.3.5).

## Doing evidence-based practice

The literature describes various ways of doing evidence-based practice, offering practical examples and tips on how to search for and appraise the evidence (usually meaning research findings). These include generic frameworks of evidence-based practice such as the guidelines provided by Sackett et al (2000) (see Box 13.1) and discipline-specific models such as Egan et al's (1998) client-centred process of evidence-based practice based upon the occupational performance process. Readers who are interested in finding out more about the practical elements of evidence-based practice can refer to the wealth of literature on the subject (e.g. see Taylor (2007); Straus (2005)).

## Barriers to evidence-based practice

Practitioners often ask, 'is evidence-based practice achievable?' Research studies have identified lack of time in particular as a persistent barrier to carrying out the steps in Box 13.1. Other identified barriers include insufficient computer resources, poor critical appraisal skills, lack of statistical knowledge, existing pressures of workload, insufficient support from colleagues and managers, complicated administrative procedures for approving new interventions, fear of challenging practices and personal reasons such as working part-time hours (Dysart and Tomlin 2002; Forsyth et al 2005; Hammond and Klompenhouwer 2005). Whilst these potential barriers are acknowledged, they are rarely insurmountable and most practitioners can take steps towards integrating an element of evidence-based practice in their work. As will be demonstrated, the integration of professional theory with evidence-based practice is one way of making the process less alien to time-pressed practitioners.

## Theory and evidence-based practice

As outlined in the introduction to this chapter, the following sections discuss four ways in which theory can and arguably should inform evidence-based practice for occupational therapists. This includes discussions around what is meant by *science*, using conceptual professional models, types of evidences and research findings.

### *The use of theory to underpin the science of evidence-based practice*

Evidence-based practice and scientific practice are often referred to as synonymous concepts and there are clear links between evidence-based practice and the generation and implementation of scientific knowledge. However terms such as *science* and *scientific* have different meanings depending upon who is using them. According to Chalmers (1999), a common-sense understanding of science is the discovery of facts via careful, unbiased processes such as experimental methods. These facts form the basis of scientific disciplines and are awarded a significant degree of prestige (from the common-sense perspective, if something is said to be *scientific* its truthfulness is usually assumed). However, as Chalmers (1999) and other authors have observed (e.g. Kuhn 1962), science is rarely this straightforward. Facts are frequently abandoned or revised and science itself is complicated by human error and changing ways of thinking. Therefore, if evidence-based practice is to be regarded as scientific practice, it is unlikely to be a straightforward process. Rather, as with other areas of science, evidence-based practice must take into account the circumstances under which facts are generated, the complex nature of human beings to whom facts are applied and the different paradigms of thought that characterise the professionals who make efforts to implement facts in practice.

In the past, occupational therapists have been advised to adapt the principles and practices of evidence-based medicine for their own use. For example, Bennett and Bennett (2000) urge therapists to adapt the process of evidence-based medicine by changing the medical concepts used within that process to concepts that are more compatible with occupational therapy (e.g. changing the label *diagnosis* to *occupational performance deficits*). However, this is only a surface consideration. Occupational therapists also need to consider the fundamental difference between the scientific philosophies underlying medicine and occupational therapy.

Broadly speaking, medicine aligns itself with positivism, a way of viewing science as a process by which unbiased methods are used to obtain objective facts about the world (similar to the common-sense view of science described by Chalmers (1999)). Consequently, the research tools of medicine are usually large-scale studies carried out in highly controlled environments (e.g. double blind randomised controlled trials).

Occupational therapy, on the other hand, is primarily concerned with the subjective experience of occupation and aligns more closely with the science of constructivism. In contrast to positivism, constructivism assumes that reality is constructed by the person experiencing it and that there are multiple realities and multiple ways of knowing (Charmaz 2000). Rather than looking for universal rules with which to understand the world, constructivists seek to understand the meanings given to events or objects by the people experiencing them. Therefore, they are more likely to use qualitative research methods such as in-depth interviews and participant observation.

However, the philosophical divide between medicine and occupational therapy is not always this simple; for example, there is obviously nothing to preclude occupational therapists from engaging in such research methods as randomised controlled trials when appropriate and doctors today are more likely to recognise the interplay of subjectivity in their work (reflected in the recent enthusiasm for reflective practice) and value the findings of qualitative research. Similarly, certain fields of occupational therapy rely heavily upon objective measurement and may benefit from quantitative evaluation (e.g. hand therapy). The distinction is also not exclusive to medicine and occupational therapy but also occurs between other academic and professional disciplines and even between different practice settings. Nevertheless, there are clear influences of differing theoretical paradigms (positivism and constructivism; see Chapter 2) underlying medicine and occupational therapy and these have implications for evidence-based practice. This is particularly so in relation to the type of evidence sought to inform professional decision-making. For example, medical professionals may be interested in the evidence offered by epidemiology (a discipline concerned with large-scale population-based studies), whereas occupational therapists may be interested in individual qualitative case studies and data from in-depth interviews. The philosophical differences are also apparent in the way that evidence-based practice is implemented. For example, medical professionals are likely to use fairly rigid procedures with proven effectiveness, whereas occupational therapists may be more flexible in their use of evidenced-based interventions as they respond to the unique occupational worlds of their clients.

### The use of an occupational therapy conceptual model in the practice of evidence-based practice

In the following discussion, the Canadian Model of Occupational Performance – CMOP-E (Townsend and Polatajko 2007) – is used to illustrate the use of conceptual professional models within evidence-based practice. Many practitioners already use an occupational therapy professional conceptual model in their work, either implicitly through their clinical reasoning process or explicitly through use of specially designed guidelines and documentation. The implementation of evidence-based practice within a theoretical framework is, therefore, suited to what may be happening already.

The potential for using the Canadian Model of Occupational Performance within evidence-based practice is extensive (see, e.g. Egan et al (1998)); however, conceptual professional models are specifically relevant to the line of enquiry or question that prompts the search for evidence in the first place. For example, a therapist using the

Canadian Model of Occupational Performance and considering a client with a physical diagnosis is driven to consider not only the characteristics of the illness or disability, but also the interactions between the illness or disability, the environment, the client's occupational performance and the client's spirituality (which may or may not have religious connotations). Such deliberations are likely to bring about questions that are far more complicated than the sort of questions driven by models of evidence-based practice interested only in diagnosis and treatment. This questioning process itself may be supported by evidence in the form of information offered by the client (what is important to him or her, what existing support is available, what are his or her occupational strengths and needs?) and research (e.g. qualitative case studies of individuals who have gone through similar experiences).

Conceptual professional models not only enable therapists to connect with the theoretical foundations of their work but they also articulate the nature of their profession (Feaver and Creek 1993). The Canadian Model of Occupational Performance (Townsend et al 1997, 2002; Townsend and Polatajko 2007) places the client at the heart of therapy, not only in terms of a human being with a diagnosis, but as a unique spiritual being. Therefore client-centred practice, although not exclusively the domain of occupational therapy, is strongly woven into the identity of therapists using this model. The therapeutic partnership between therapists and clients, as a mechanism of client-centred practice, invites both parties to contribute their expertise to the problem-solving process. Evidence-based practice can be interpreted as the therapist's commitment to this partnership by drawing attention to as many options for therapy as possible together with information about their effectiveness and potential risk. Clients then contribute their *expertise* by critiquing this evidence in terms of its suitability to their particular circumstances and by providing additional information (such as information about existing coping strategies). In an ideal situation, therapists and clients critically appraise this information together in order to arrive at a decision about intervention (Reagon et al 2008).

Finally, because conceptual professional models illustrate particular beliefs held by occupational therapists, they determine how practitioners interpret evidence. For example, the Canadian Model of Occupational Performance (Townsend et al 1997, 2002; Townsend and Polatajko 2007) expresses a theory about the interrelationship between the individual, the environment and occupation and that change in one area, instigates change in all three areas. Therefore, occupational therapists using this model will make sense of evidence in light of its tenets. For example, working in such a way would make therapists using the model approach a research article describing the effectiveness of two interventions in a clinical trial as follows: If the interventions described involve modifications to one component of the triad (e.g. the environment), how will this impact upon the other components (e.g. the individual and their occupations) and what are the implications of this for therapy?

### The use of theory in seeking the evidence base

Once a therapist has identified the issues that might be pertinent to a particular case and formulated questions, the search for evidence begins (note that, as is frequently the case in qualitative research and reflecting their scientific paradigm, occupational therapists might identify general issues to explore rather than precise questions). One immediate source of information is the therapist's theoretical knowledge about occupation and its transformative effects on health and well-being. This may be complemented and extended by reading the occupational science literature. Occupational science – the 'rigorous study of humans as occupational beings' (Wilcock 2001, p. 413) – offers an alternative to traditional knowledge bases such as medicine and sociology by its systematic exploration of occupation.

There are two other major sources of information that therapists can refer to in their pursuit of evidence: research and the client. Research is perhaps the most obvious resource, often referred to exclusively, in discussions about evidence-based practice. Various models of research utilisation are also offered in the occupational therapy literature (e.g. Bennett and Bennett 2000) and are comparative to Sackett et al's (2000) view of evidence-based practice. There has also been a wide debate about how to incorporate research into practice, including discussions about how to bridge the research-practice gap effectively, and what constitutes the best type of research evidence (sometimes illustrated by evidence hierarchies). The *paradigm war* between quantitative and qualitative research, although settled in some spheres, is unfortunately still alive in many practice settings. However, regardless of debates about robustness, and the paradigmatic view, the research methods chosen should be those that promise to best answer the research questions. In occupational therapy, relevant research questions are often, but not exclusively, qualitative in nature. As the Canadian Model of Occupational Performance (Townsend et al 1997, 2002; Townsend and Polatajko 2007) emphasises, occupational therapists are concerned with the spiritual, intellectual and emotional aspects of human beings, as well as values and morals that are often beyond the observable aspects of performance. Qualitative research methods, with their emphasis on the exploration of the subjective, are particularly congruent with these concerns. Finally, Cusick (2001, p. 110) warns of the danger of not incorporating qualitative evidence into occupational therapy decision-making:

> If we do not do this [use qualitative research] we may find, to our great loss, that in the process of fostering evidence-based practitioners, we suffer the unintended consequence of sidelining important dimensions of our practice, thus losing the innovation and insight of our qualitative research, and unintentionally nurturing a deterministic practice, thereby furthering the dominance of biomedical approaches to human health.

Clients form the second major source of evidence for occupational therapists and, unlike theories derived from research, are immediately relevant and accessible. Clients offer information about their experiences of occupational therapy intervention, health conditions, social circumstances, past and present occupations, value and belief systems and perceptions of life in general. Given the client-centred philosophy of occupational therapy, it seems absurd to regard this type of information as secondary to more recognised evidence such as research. In many areas of practice, gathering information from clients and others involved in the case (relatives, friends, colleagues) is a primary component of the problem-solving process. Questions asked could provide access to information about clients' health conditions, histories, degrees of insight, levels of independence, desired goals and current coping strategies (government literature in the United Kingdom encourages clients to become *experts* in managing their conditions (Department of Health 2001)). Clients may also offer important information about the perceived suitability and success of a particular intervention that can be combined with outcome measurements and theories from research. However, as with all information gathering, there may be circumstances in which clients cannot clearly articulate their thoughts, in which case therapists need to be creative.

### The relationship between theory and research evidence

Regardless of the organisation in which they work, health care practitioners inevitably make choices that impact upon finite resources such as money, staff, time and technology. Even clients who pay for their health care are limited by the services available to them. Evidence-based practice plays an increasing role in deciding which services are available and which are not by using research to determine their cost-effectiveness and enabling policy-makers and managers to make informed decisions about which services to support. Today, there is a real danger that under-researched interventions will cease to be purchased in favour of well-researched alternatives or, worse still, nothing at all. Therefore, occupational therapists have a responsibility to develop research capacity as a matter of urgency.

However, whilst it is tempting to develop a research evidence base with strong statistical power, research needs to reflect occupational therapy's values. As has been argued, scientific research is not designed and conducted in a theoretical vacuum; rather researchers are influenced by their prior knowledge and experience, philosophical perspectives (including their understanding of science) and existing theories (Chalmers 1999). These influence the research questions asked, the research approach adopted and the methods of data collection and analysis. For example, an occupational therapist viewing data for a particular research project will *see* things differently to a psychologist or a nurse viewing the same dataset. These different ways of *seeing* are not necessarily in competition but bring different perspectives to a phenomenon. Nevertheless, occupational therapists should not undertake research projects simply to maintain the status quo; rather, the outcomes of research should be used to test, support, and modify existing theories and to build new theories.

## Conclusion

Evidence-based practice is an imperative in the modern world as demand for health care rises, and the quality and cost-effectiveness of services are increasingly scrutinised. However, evidence-based practice, although often used as a generic term, means different things to different groups of professionals. This reflects the fact that professional identities are shaped by diverse theories and philosophies.

This chapter has demonstrated the interrelationship between evidence-based practice and theory for occupational therapists. Firstly, it explored the underlying science of occupational therapy, which is more akin to constructivism than positivism. This influences the ways in which occupational therapists understand and carry out evidence-based practice, the type of evidence they look for and the sorts of research questions they seek to answer. Secondly, it considered the use of an occupational therapy professional conceptual model within evidence-based practice, demonstrating how this guides the process of evidence-based practice by articulating occupational therapy's theories and values, for example in how therapists interpret evidence. Thirdly, it demonstrated how theory focuses the search for evidence by directing therapists towards the occupational science literature, relevant research data and client-specific evidence. Fourthly, it demonstrated that the process of research, an integral part of evidence-based practice, is determined by the theories of occupational therapy such as its understanding of science. Finally, it argued that research needs to be developed by occupational therapists to support, challenge and extend their theories about occupation and the effectiveness of their interventions.

# References

Bennett, S. and Bennett, J.W. (2000) The process of evidence-based practice in occupational therapy: informing clinical decisions. *Australian Occupational Therapy Journal* 47, 171–180.

Chalmers, A.F. (1999) *What is this Thing Called Science?*, 3rd edn. Buckingham: Open University Press.

Charmaz, K. (2000) Grounded Theory: Objectivist and Constructivist Methods. In: *Handbook of Qualitative Research*, eds N.K. Denzin and Y.S. Lincoln, 2nd edn, pp. 509–535. Thousand Oaks: Sage.

College of Occupational Therapists (2010) *Code of Ethics and Professional Conduct*. London: College of Occupational Therapists.

Creswell, J.W. (2011) *Designing and Conducting Mixed Methods Research*. London: Sage.

Cusick, A. (2001) OZ OT EBP 21C: Australian Occupational Therapy, evidence-based practice and the 21st century. *Australian Occupational Therapy Journal* 48(3), 102–117.

Department of Health (2001) *The Expert Patient: A New Approach to Chronic Disease Management for the 21st Century*. London: Department of Health.

Dysart, A.M. and Tomlin, G.S. (2002) Factors related to evidence-based practice among US occupational therapy clinicians. *The American Journal of Occupational Therapy* 65(2), 189–196.

Egan, M., Dubouloz, C.J., von Zweck, C. and Vallerand, J. (1998) The client-centred evidence-based practice of occupational therapy. *Canadian Journal of Occupational Therapy* 65(3), 136–143.

Feaver, S. and Creek, J. (1993) Models of practice in occupational therapy. Part 2: what use are they? *British Journal of Occupational Therapy* 56(2), 59–62.

Forsyth, K., Summerfield Mann, L. and Kielhofner, G. (2005) Scholarship of practice: making occupation-focused, theory-driven, evidence-based practice a reality. *British Journal of Occupational Therapy* 68(6), 260–268.

Gray, J.A.M. (2001) *Evidence-Based Healthcare*, 2nd edn. Edinburgh: Churchill Livingstone.

Greenhalgh, T. (2002) Intuition and evidence – uneasy bedfellows? *British Journal of General Practice* 52(478), 395–400.

Hammond, A. and Klompenhouwer, P. (2005) Getting evidence into practice: implementing a Behavioural Joint Protection Education Programme for people with rheumatoid arthritis. *British Journal of Occupational Therapy* 68(1), 25–33.

Kuhn, T.S. (1962) *The Structure of Scientific Revolutions*. Chicago: University of Chicago Press.

Reagon, C., Bellin, W. and Boniface, G. (2008) Reconfiguring evidence-based practice for occupational therapists. *International Journal of Therapy and Rehabilitation* 15(10), 428–435.

Sackett, D., Rosenberg, W.M., Gray, J.A.M., Haynes, R.B. and Richardson, W.S. (1996) Evidence based medicine: what it is and what it isn't. *British Medical Journal* 312, 71–72.

Sackett, D.L., Straus, S.E., Richardson, W.S., Rosenberg, W.M. and Haynes, R.B. (2000) *Evidence-Based Medicine: How to Practice and Teach EBM*. Edinburgh: Churchill Livingstone.

Straus, S.E., Richardson, W.S., Glasziou, P. and Haynes, R.B. (2005) Evidence-Based Medicine: How to Practice and Teach EBM, 3rd edn. Edinburgh: Churchill Livingstone.

Taylor, M.C. (2007) *Evidence-Based Practice for Occupational Therapists*, 2nd edn. Oxford: Blackwell Science.

Townsend, E., Stanton, S., Law, M., Polatajko, H., Baptiste, S., Thompson-Franson, T., Kramer, C., Swedlove, F., Brintnell, S. and Campanile, L. (1997) *Enabling Occupation: An Occupational Therapy Perspective*. Ottawa, ON: CAOT ACE.

Townsend, E., Stanton, S., Law, M., Polatajko, H., Baptiste, S., Thompson-Franson, T., Kramer, C., Swedlove, F., Brintnell, S. and Campanile, L. (2002) *Enabling Occupation: An Occupational Therapy Perspective*. Ottawa, ON: CAOT ACE.

Townsend, E.A. and Polatajko, H.J. (2007) *Enabling Occupation II: Advancing an Occupational Therapy Vision for Health, Well-Being & Justice through Occupation*. Ottawa, ON: CAOT ACE.

Trinder, L. (2000) Introduction: the context of evidence-based practice. In: *Evidence-Based Practice: A Critical Appraisal*, eds L. Trinder and R. Reynolds, pp. 1–16. Oxford: Blackwell Science.

Wilcock, A.A. (2001) Occupational science: the key to broadening horizons. *British Journal of Occupational Therapy* 64(8), 412–417.

## Further reading

Straus, S.E., Richardson, W.S., Glasziou, P. and Haynes, R.B. (2005) *Evidence-Based Medicine: How to Practice and Teach EBM*, 3rd edn. Edinburgh: Churchill Livingstone.

Taylor, M.C. (2007) *Evidence-Based Practice for Occupational Therapists*, 2nd edn. Oxford: Blackwell Science.

Trinder, L. and Reynolds, R. (eds) (2000) *Evidence-Based Practice: A Critical Appraisal*. Oxford: Blackwell Science.

# Chapter 14

# Occupational science and occupational therapy: a contemporary relationship

*Jill Riley*

---

**Key points**

- The historical relationship between occupational science as an academic discipline and occupational therapy remains strong
- Occupational science can enhance occupational therapists' understanding of occupation from different perspectives
- Occupation as a complex and multi-faceted phenomenon, its forms and domain require understanding as a prerequisite to analysing an individual's occupational performance

---

## Introduction

As an academic discipline, occupational science is concerned with the study of human occupation, in other words, what people do on a day-to-day basis in the context of their natural environment, community, society and culture. As a relatively new discipline, occupational science emerged in the late twentieth century from a close relationship with occupational therapy (University of Southern California 2009). In the twenty-first century it continues to grow and develop as a discipline in its own right. In this chapter, I examine today's relationship between occupational science and occupational therapy, by exploring how occupational science theory can now inform contemporary occupational therapy practice. The discussion includes an analysis of different definitions and perspectives on occupation and how it is conceptualised in practice through the use of an occupational therapy professional model and occupational analysis.

## Occupational science: an emerging discipline

Occupational science officially emerged as an academic discipline in 1989 at the University of Southern California, with the launch of a doctoral programme. Its purpose at

---

*Using Occupational Therapy Theory in Practice*, First Edition. Edited by Gail Boniface and Alison Seymour.
© 2012 Blackwell Publishing Ltd. Published 2012 by Blackwell Publishing Ltd.

the time was to provide a scientific base for occupational therapy practice (University of Southern California 2009; Pierce et al 2010) through research into the different aspects, components and complexities of human occupation. As a discipline that focuses on the centrality of occupation to humans, occupational science now draws on a wide range of inter-disciplinary fields, including anthropology, geography, sociology, psychology, bio-sciences, education and arts. Throughout its short history, the discipline has developed a unique knowledge base relating to human occupation that other disciplines can draw on as well as continue to inform occupational therapy practice.

During the last two decades, academic centres and societies for the study of occupational science have developed in North America, Australia and the United Kingdom. More recently, the International Society for Occupational Science (ISOS) has begun to facilitate an international network of individuals and institutions that are committed to occupation-focused research and education and to promoting occupation for health and community development (ISOS 2007, p. 1). By 2017, ISOS hopes that the knowledge gained from occupational science research will be 'translated into practices and policies that enhance everyday living for individuals, families and communities' (p. 2). The society also hopes that occupational therapists worldwide will incorporate occupational science into education and practice.

As an academic discipline, occupational science has its own peer-reviewed journal, the *Journal of Occupational Science*, which promotes the study of humans as occupational beings. The journal, established in 1993, publishes occupational science research and provides a forum for discussion and debate about issues relating to the study of human occupation. A stock take of insights into the study of occupation up to 2000, from this journal and occupational therapy journals (Hocking 2000a), pointed to an assumed relationship between occupation and health, probably arising from occupational science's close alliance with occupational therapy. The relationship between occupation and health is reinforced by Anne Wilcock's occupational theory of human nature, which asserts that humans have an innate need to engage in purposeful occupation and that this is related to health and survival (Wilcock 1993, 1998). Others have related perceptions of health and well-being to the satisfaction and meaning derived from occupation (Nelson 1988; Yerxa 1998). Well-being, coming from engaging in meaningful occupation, was also seen as contributing to a sense of self and identity (Reynolds 1997; Christiansen 1999). Hocking's review of the literature also identified the 'culturally embedded nature of occupation', together with its temporal nature, subjective and social meanings (Hocking 2000a, p. 64).

A more recent systematic analysis of the occupational science literature from 1996 to 2006 (Glover 2009) evidenced a growth in the discipline's body of knowledge, emanating from theoretical work and empirically based research. Glover found that a substantial body of occupational science research was conducted with adults who did not have disabilities; as she puts it, 'this points to the health of occupational science as a discipline related to, but not dependent on, occupational therapy' (p. 100). In Glover's view, because of the strong relationship between occupational science and occupational therapy, and the unique centrality of occupation to both fields, occupational science research can inform therapeutic practice and draw questions from it. In turn, Glover's review revealed that a large proportion of occupational scientists were also occupational therapists, an indication of the continuing strength of the relationship between the two fields. Indeed, Clarke (2006) described the relationship as 'symbiotic' (p. 172); in her view 'one will not survive without the other' (p. 173). However, Glover found that occupational scientists also came from other disciplines such as anthropology, psychology, sociology or neuro-science, albeit in small numbers. This supports the view that perspectives on occupation from fields other that occupational therapy can enrich the discipline, which is now developing as an inter-disciplinary science and a discipline in its own right (Glover 2009), something which in Clarke's (2006) view, needs to be strengthened.

A further and equally insightful study identifying the research patterns in the first 5 years of presentations to the Society for the Study of Occupation (SSO): the United States revealed two primary theoretical perspectives relating to the usefulness of occupational science research to occupational therapy and social science theories and methods (Pierce et al 2010). Pierce et al perceived 'a tension between perspectives emanating from the needs of occupational therapy versus the needs for developing social perspectives on occupation' (p. 207). They found that in the United States the relationship between occupational science and occupational therapy remains strong, even though the majority of studies were conducted with adults without disabilities. They point to presentations of occupation-based practice research as the clearest examples of the strength of this relationship, and found that within some, information flowed from practice to theory rather than the other way round (Pierce et al 2010). This contradicts the view that theory should underpin practice; but on the other hand, it is a reminder that occupational science's roots were practice – based in the first place. It also suggests that research questions that lead to the generation of occupational science theory can come from practice. So far it is evident that a relationship between occupational science and occupational therapy is very much alive, but Pierce et al's (2010) study raised a further pertinent question when considering the future of occupational science as a discipline, which will be addressed in the next section.

## Is occupational science research too individualistic?

Occupational therapists naturally focus on occupation from an individual's perspective. Their concerns lie with individuals' occupational performance, function and meanings whilst taking into account their sociocultural environment and how they might adapt to problems encountered. Professional occupational therapy models help therapists to understand and *frame* these issues within the umbrella of occupational theory (see Chapter 3) and occupational analysis is a tool for breaking down and analysing the components of occupational performance. It naturally follows that from an occupational therapy perspective, the study of occupation should be individualistic. On the other hand, however, knowledge generated about occupation from an individualistic perspective alone can be regarded as too narrow to elicit a holistic understanding of occupation as a multi-dimensional and complex phenomenon. Jarman (2004), for example, explored inter-disciplinary perspectives on definitions of occupation; moving from occupational therapy's individualistic view of occupation to a social science perspective on occupation as work. The latter takes into account how occupational structures evolve together with the meaning this has for society and social inequality. In other words, a social science perspective views occupation in a broader context.

Others have also argued for a contextual view of occupation, and in 2006 an interesting debate arose in the *Journal of Occupational Science*. Dickie et al (2006) proposed that occupation is transactional and extends beyond individual experience encompassing a 'social, physical and cultural context' (p. 85). This view suggests that it is important to consider the relationship between the individual, the occupation and the environment in context. In contrast, Barber (2006) emphasised a 'first-person perspective' (p. 94) and how individuals experience occupation and the environmental-contextual factors for themselves. There is a fundamental issue here in terms of how occupation is defined and researched; Pierce et al (2010) argue that moving away from a predominantly individualistic approach would require a radical change in how occupation is conceptualised, researched and reported. There is, it seems, a growing tension between occupational science as a discipline that serves the needs of occupational therapy on the one hand and occupational science as an inter-disciplinary field that can develop knowledge and theories for application in wider contexts on the other. Ann Wilcock's intention was that her occupational theory of health (1998, 2006) had, and still has, the potential to inform public health initiatives and ultimately policy development, although she acknowledges that her early work was largely adopted by occupational therapists. As the occupational science discipline grows and new perspectives on occupation develop through research (e.g. the impact of the social and political environment on occupational engagement (Laliberte-Rudman 2002), occupational alienation, disfranchisement, risk and deprivation (French 2002), occupational justice and injustice (Jakobsen 2004; Mernar 2006)), the greater the science's potential to contribute to inter-disciplinary contexts. However, it can, and should, continue to inform occupational therapy as one of those disciplines. So, working from the assumption that occupational science will continue to inform occupational therapy, and that the use of theory in practice is occupational therapy's and not occupational science's concern; how can occupational therapists make use of occupational science knowledge and theory?

## From theory to practice

In Chapters 2 and 3 of this book, it has been asserted that as professionals, occupational therapists should harness theory and be able to translate this into use in practice. Theories of occupation can be considered as the profession's *espoused* theories and models of occupational therapy are proposed as both a theoretical base and a tool for practice (see Chapter 3). In addition, occupational analysis is acknowledged as a core skill for occupational therapy practice. The following sections discuss how the use of occupational therapy professional models and occupational analysis might lead occupational therapists to make use of occupational science knowledge and theory.

# Occupational science theory and occupational therapy models

The fundamental difference between theories of occupation and occupational therapy models is that the former conceptualise and describe the complexity of human occupation for individuals and in context, whereas models are theoretical definitions of the profession (see Chapter 3); they come from practice and guide practice. Chapter 3 offers a definition and overview of the different occupational therapy professional models; here I intend to draw out some of the aspects of models that should lead occupational therapists towards occupational science in order to gain a greater depth of understanding of human occupation.

Occupation is, as we have seen in previous chapters, a central concept of occupational therapy professional models, which also recognise the relationship between occupation and health. Turpin and Iwama (2011) propose that occupational therapy professional models have been influenced by three models of health: biomedical, biopyschosocial and socioecological. The biomedical model emphasises a mechanistic approach to restoring health and consequently a somewhat reductionist, therapeutic use of activity, or even tasks to improve performance skills. The second, biopsychosocial model takes a systems approach, where social and psychological issues are considered alongside biological concerns. This model of health has, to date, strongly influenced the development of occupational therapy theory and models of occupational therapy (Turpin and Iwama 2011). However, the recently revised edition of the Canadian Model of Occupational Performance – CMOP-E (Townsend and Polatajko 2007) is entrenched in a belief that occupation is a determinant of health and well-being and fits more closely with a socioecological model, which takes account of health determinants. *Enabling Occupation II* (Townsend and Polatajko 2007) encompasses occupational engagement and relates occupation, health and well-being to justice. It also recognises that occupation is not always health promoting, in that the idiosyncratic and sometimes harmful nature of occupation, for example drug-taking or vandalism, can be detrimental to both the individual and society.

Although models of occupational therapy offer broad definitions of occupation and seek to categorise them from an individual's perspective and identify influencing factors, they do not offer any substantial detail about the nature of occupation or the complexity of the contexts of occupational engagement and performance. This is not their purpose, but they can assist occupational therapists in identifying aspects of occupational engagement and the influencing environmental, sociocultural and temporal factors that require further investigation. The following example illustrates how the most recent Canadian Model of Occupational Performance and Engagement (CMOP-E) (Townsend and Polatajko 2007) might assist therapists in identifying theories of occupation to underpin practice.

> John, now in his early 50s, has worked for most of his adult life as a self-employed builder. He is currently unable to work due to back problems that have resulted in chronic pain. John divorced his wife several years ago and now lives with his elderly mother. John was known

by his colleagues in the building trade and by his clients as a highly skilled carpenter and creative problem-solver. He is also a skilled wood-carver and made hand-crafted furniture in his spare time. He occasionally took commissions, exhibited and sold his work. John's inability to work and continue making furniture resulting from his chronic pain and his concentration on caring for himself and his mother have also made him depressed and anxious about the future.

The CMOP-E recognises John as a spiritual being with the potential to identify and choose the occupations he wants to engage in. The model emphasises the dynamic relationship between occupational performance, engagement and environmental contexts that change over time and across the lifespan (Townsend and Polatajko 2007). Spiritually, John strongly values his craftsmanship and his ability to create original objects from wood as a raw material, something he is anxious to return to. John also valued the independence and autonomy that came from being self-employed. John might choose to engage in his valued occupations, but illness and the resulting social circumstances have taken away his ability to do so. John's only source of income now comes from welfare benefits and this has also impacted on how society perceives him. John, an only child, now cares for and lives with his elderly mother, who has come to rely on him for help with activities of daily living.

Because John is now living with his mother, his environment has also changed on physical, social and institutional levels (Townsend and Polatajko 2007). Physically he has less room to store the materials and the equipment he needs to engage in any form of wood work. He has moved to a different community and needs to rebuild his social networks and institutionally his occupational performance is influenced by his need to claim state benefits and support needs in terms of returning to work.

By focussing on John's occupational performance and engagement, and seeing him as a spiritual being with personal values, the CMOP-E assists us in identifying specific aspects of John's occupational engagement that require further understanding. It leads to the generation of occupationally focussed questions (listed later). The model also takes into account the broader contexts that influence John's occupational engagement and performance. These include, for example, institutional factors such as the social welfare system on which John now relies for income and support; the sociocultural changes arising from growing numbers of older people in Western societies, which means that John is still caring for his mother whilst approaching older adulthood himself. There are also issues relating to gender and occupation that are socially constructed and might impact on John's identity and sense of self as his occupational roles change.

The following occupationally focussed questions arise from using CMOP-E as a framework to understand John as an occupational being:

1. How does occupational engagement impact on John's sense of self and identity?
2. How do John's current circumstances affect his balance of occupations?
3. What impacts on John's occupational choice and participation?

Such questions lead to an exploration of knowledge and theory embedded in occupational science. Broadly, the answer to the first question requires an understanding of occupational identity, the second occupational balance and choice, and the third the impact of occupational deprivation and justice. In later sections, I will relate these concepts to John in more detail, but to fully comprehend this relationship, an understanding of the nature of John's occupations is also necessary. Occupational analysis, a core skill of occupational therapy, offers occupational therapists a way of understanding and analysing the components of occupation. The Section 'Understanding and analysing occupation' offers a critique of occupational analysis frameworks and questions how much they contribute to an understanding of occupation.

## Understanding and analysing occupation

Occupational analysis is defined by Townsend and Polatajko (2007) as 'a form of assessment focussed on occupation' (p. 369) and they consider that an analysis of the components of occupation requires competency. This is unsurprising in view of the complex and multi-faceted nature of occupation. Various frameworks have been developed to assist occupational therapists with the task and these vary, both in complexity and in their use of terminology. Here, I will concentrate on three different ways of understanding and analysing occupation described in the occupational therapy literature. The first, put forward by Hagedorn (1995, 1997), takes a hierarchical view of occupation, breaking it down into activities and tasks. The second, developed by Brienes (1995) proposes that occupational or activity analysis corresponds to a systems model. The third, Nelson (1988, 1994) proposed a conceptual framework to assist therapists' understanding of occupation that is concerned with the relationship between occupational form and occupational performance. Nelson's framework for therapeutic occupation was developed further by Nelson and Jepson-Thomas (2003).

Hagedorn's (1995) view of occupation is as 'a structured form of human endeavour' (p. 84) that is longitudinal, organising time and effort. In her view, because occupations are lived, or experienced, they are not performed. Occupations comprise activities, which 'take place on specific occasions, for a finite period and for a specific purpose' and tasks are a component of activity (Hagedorn 1997, p. 25). For Hagedorn, occupational analysis should take account of the individual's participation and the nature of the occupation. The individual must decide whether their occupational participation is categorised as work, leisure or self-care. Because Hagedorn defines occupations as lived experience, and the activities that contribute to the occupation are performed, analysis takes place at this level. It involves breaking down the activity into components (tasks); identifying sequences; the types of performance required; degrees of complexity; and the social and environmental needs. If this form of analysis is applied to John's occupation of furniture making, then he must categorise his participation. For John, making furniture might be mainly a leisure pursuit, but with an element of work and even *self-care* if the term is used to encompass psychological and spiritual caring for the self as well as physical aspects. (Such differing possible categorisations demonstrating that indeed occupational participation rarely fall into neat categories). Then, furniture making must be broken down into component activities and further into tasks, which can then be analysed in terms of the specific physical, cognitive and interactional skills required to achieve them.

Hagedorn (1997) also refers to environmental analysis as necessary to ascertain the effect of the environment on the occupation and the participant. This includes the content, which in John's case includes his working space, equipment and tools; the demand that is the psychological, cultural and social impacts on performance and finally adaptation: how the environment might be changed to enhance performance opportunities. Hagedorn offers a relatively straightforward and somewhat systematic approach to analysing *activities* and *tasks*, which takes into account the environment where these are performed. Arguably, it offers occupational therapists a means of understanding the components of an occupation by breaking down its complexity, rather than the nature of an occupation as a whole.

Brienes (1995) also refers to *activity* analysis, describing it as 'a complex and extensive process that examines all the effects that activities can potentially provide, simultaneously and sequentially' (p. 26).

The process is complex because there is a relationship between different performance dimensions that cannot be seen in isolation. Brienes describes the relationships elicited through activity as the coming together of egocentric, exocentric and consensual elements. Meaningful activities integrate these elements resulting in 'wholesomeness' (Brienes 1995, p. 26), conceptualised as health and well-being. An analysis of John's furniture making using this approach would bring together the physical and mental abilities that John needs to accomplish the tasks involved in making (the egocentric elements) with the external (exocentric) elements such as the tools and equipment, space and time required. There may also be consensual elements if John needs to communicate with suppliers to obtain materials and equipment for example, or chooses to sell his work to others. John's well-being or *wholesomeness* comes from the integration of these elements in this meaningful activity.

The theory underpinning Breines's approach to analysing activity takes into account the historical development of occupation and its evolution over time. Drawing on the work of philosopher John Dewey, Breines (1995) refers to this as occupational genesis, which grounds the 'meaningfulness of activity' and its sociocultural relevance (p. 3). This places activity in a cultural and temporal context, recognising that relevance and meaning change over time. In twenty-first century Western society, for example, it is no longer necessary to make furniture by hand for purely utilitarian purposes; it is mass-produced. Today, hand-crafted furniture has a sociocultural value as an art form, because of its uniqueness. It might also represent cultural traditions, a link with the past. For John, making furniture was also a form of self-expression. Working creatively by hand and exercising his skills by engaging with raw materials contributed to his physical, psychological and spiritual well-being.

The third occupational analysis framework I wish to discuss is a conceptual framework for therapeutic occupation, developed by Nelson (1988, 1994) and Nelson and Jepson-Thomas (2003). This framework conceptualises occupation as the relationship between occupational form and occupational performance (Nelson 1988). Occupational form is defined as 'an objective set of circumstances, external to the person, that elicits, guides, or structures the person's occupational performance' (Nelson 1994, p. 11). Performance is the 'doing', the action involved in carrying out occupation. In other words, occupation involves a form, or format, that is performed (Nelson 1988). In this framework, it is necessary to understand not just the doing or action involved in performance, in other words the activity level, but the entire context of occupation, that is the occupational form. For Nelson, occupational form has both physical and socio-cultural aspects. It also has meaning for the performing individual who will interpret it in different ways. Nelson also takes into account the unique developmental structure that individuals bring to the occupational form and their purpose, the resulting outcome of occupational performance (Nelson 1994).

By using Nelson's occupational analysis conceptual framework to understand John's occupation of furniture making, one can gain an in-depth understanding of furniture making as an occupational form by separating it from performance in the first instance. Nelson and Jepson-Thomas (2003) describe occupational form as objective, a phenomenon that can be studied in its own right. The physical components such as the materials, equipment and tools, suppliers, workshop space and time, for example are similar to Brienes' (1995) exocentric elements and can be identified in Hagedorn's (1997) environmental analysis. Nelson also considers the social and cultural influences that have an impact on occupational form. These might include society's view of hand-craft in the context of British culture, and how culture has influenced the development of furniture making in contemporary society, things that Breines takes account of in her theory of occupational genesis, but are perhaps less evident in Hagedorn's hierarchical view of analysis.

Nelson talks about occupational form as having pre-existing structures that guide performance (Nelson 1988). These can be considered as habitual practices that are embedded in tradition, in that they are accepted and transmissible patterns of human action (Shils 1981). Arguably, all occupational forms incorporate traditional patterns of action that are socioculturally determined, they develop in a historical context (Riley 2011). Making a piece of furniture as a process involves multiple patterns of action that the maker engages in from design to completing a finished product. If separated out, each could be described as an activity and analysed as such, but occupational form must be understood as a complex unity of different dimensions (Nelson and Jepson-Thomas 2003) that is not static, but changes and evolves over time.

From an occupational science perspective, furniture making in common with other craft-oriented occupations encompasses a set of inter-related practices with common elements that are socially, culturally and historically constructed (Riley 2011). As a whole, it can be conceptualised as an occupational domain or sphere of action (Dickie 2003; Riley 2009, 2011), an interactive system with its own symbolic rules, procedures, specific skills and knowledge (Csikszentmihalyi 1996). Making furniture in itself is diverse, and different kinds of furniture making have different occupational forms, albeit with common elements. These are encompassed in the occupational domain, and individuals' actions and creativity dynamically contribute to its evolution.

In summary, analysing and breaking down occupation in a way that takes into account its multi-faceted nature and context is undoubtedly complex. Hagedorn (1997) offers a hierarchical approach for analysing individual's performance at an activity level, which takes into account the environment, but does not lead to a contextual understanding of occupation. Brienes (1995) accounts for complexity by taking an interactive systems approach and Nelson presents a conceptual framework that brings together occupational form, performance and meaning. Furthermore, an understanding of occupation in the context of an occupational domain offers a foundation for fully understanding occupational forms (Riley 2011), human action and analysing occupational performance. It also provides a context for understanding the meaning of occupation for individuals, how it impacts on their identity, ability to balance and choose the occupations they engage in. In the following sections, I return to the occupationally focussed questions listed in the preceding text and address them with reference to occupational science theory.

## Occupational identity

The first question generated from the use of CMOP-E (Townsend and Polatajko 2007) related to how John's occupational engagement impacts on his identity. A sense of self and personal fulfilment coming from engaging in particular occupations that are personally constructed, valued and have meaning is a part of occupational identity. For John, these included making furniture and being a self-employed builder. They contributed to his sense of self and personal identity; things that he has lost through occupational disruption.

From an occupational science perspective, we become who we are through what we do (Christiansen 2004). In other words, our occupational experiences and motivation to engage in particular occupations shapes our sense of self, personal and social identity. Active doing contributes to *becoming* who we are and is intimately connected with a sense of *being*, our essence and what is distinctive about us (Wilcock 1999; 2006). John became a wood carver and furniture maker by actively engaging in making and mastering the domain's skills. This came from an intrinsic drive to do something well and for its own sake (Nelson 1994; Sennett 2008); it was a fundamental part of his sense of *being*, his spirituality. John's sense of self and his social identity are also represented in the objects he makes (Hocking 2000b), which have a social and cultural value. For John, being a furniture maker with a sense of self, personal and social identity has been disrupted by illness and social circumstances. As a consequence, his occupational balance, sense of control and ability to choose which occupations to engage in are also disrupted.

## Occupational balance, choice and control

Occupational balance is a dynamic and changing process and imbalance occurs when occupations are incompatible and there is a lack of opportunity to engage in chosen occupations (Backman 2010). It is a central tenet of occupational therapy because of its impact on a client's health, well-being and satisfaction (Westhorp 2003), although it has, in the past, been poorly understood (Reed and Sanderson 1999). Indeed Wada et al (2010) argue that there is still a lack of conceptual clarity. They identify different occupational perspectives of balance that come from four different theoretical bases. The first takes account of the amount of time allocated to different occupations and how this impacts on health and well-being. The second is concerned with congruence and the extent to which occupations reflect an individual's beliefs, values and aspirations; the third, role fulfilment, includes occupational competency and ability to perform occupations and the fourth, compatibility and the extent to which an individual's occupations are in harmony. In terms of time allocation, John now spends most of his time caring for himself and his mother at the expense of the occupations that he values most and that reflect his beliefs and aspirations. He is unable to fully exercise his occupational competency and for him, his occupations lack harmony.

Taking an occupational perspective of health, Wilcock (2006) believes that imbalance occurs 'because people's engagement in occupation fails to meet either their natural health requirements for physical, social and mental exercise or rest or their unique doing, being and becoming needs' (p. 170). From this perspective, John no longer has a balance of occupations that meet his requirements and his illness has inevitably impacted on his choice of occupations. Nagle et al (2002) describe how illness can force people to 'abandon valued occupations and aspirations' (p. 75), so can John still exercise occupational choice?

Occupational choices are also governed by opportunities, personal and social circumstances and resources, all of which have changed for John. This is compounded by Western society's changing demographic profile and the expectation that he will care for his elderly mother as he grows older himself. This has also impacted on John's balance of occupations, which have by necessity become more self-care oriented, and consequently his ability to exercise occupational choice. The subsequent effects on his occupational engagement lead to further, more contextual issues relating to occupational deprivation and justice.

## Occupational deprivation and justice

Occupational deprivation is the result of external factors that inhibit occupational choice and engagement in the long term. These include environmental, social, cultural, institutional and political influences (Whiteford 2004; Townsend and Polatajko 2007). It was identified through the use of CMOP-E (Townsend and Polatajko 2007) that John's immediate environment has changed and he now has less room for the equipment and materials he needs for wood turning and making furniture. His chronic pain has impacted on his occupational performance resulting in a loss of valued productive roles and income from self-employment. As a consequence, John has to rely on state benefits, which has a further and profound effect on his occupational engagement, identity and choice. Indeed, Whiteford (2004) identifies lack of employment as one of the major contributors to occupational deprivation in the twenty-first century. Occupational deprivation can, in turn, lead to social isolation as a result of the loss of opportunity for social contact that meaningful occupation can give. John's move to a different community adds to this. Occupational deprivation together with John's occupational imbalance that has resulted from a lack of engagement in meaningful productive and valued leisure occupations at the expense of a concentration on a caring role can be seen as an outcome of occupational injustice (Townsend and Wilcock 2004). As a concept, occupational justice suggests the right to engage in meaningful occupation, to participate in occupations that promote health and social inclusion and to make occupational choices and equal rights to participate in a range of occupations, taking into account the cultural context (Townsend and Wilcock 2004; Smith and Hilton 2008). The political context is also important, where changes in government policy and legislations affect individuals' rights to work or claim benefits, for example. Townsend and Polatajko (2007) point out that the occupational therapy profession is concerned to ensure that 'people have access to opportunities and resources to participate in culturally defined, health-building occupations' (p. 80) and that 'occupational therapists have the skills to reflect on situations causing occupational injustices and work to change them' (p. 81). This necessitates an understanding and appreciation of the underlying concepts and how these impact on occupational engagement.

## Conclusion

An overview of the history and development of occupational science as an academic discipline reveals a strong and enduring relationship with occupational therapy where the concept of occupation is central to both. As occupational science continues to develop as an inter-disciplinary field, occupation is being researched and understood from different theoretical perspectives, taking into account not only an individualistic view that is the primary concern of occupational therapy but also an understanding of occupation in sociocultural and political contexts. This strengthens occupational science as a field that can continue to inform occupational therapy as one of many disciplines. However, the use of theory in practice is occupational therapy's concern. I have illustrated how a contemporary occupational therapy model, CMOP-E, can assist occupational therapists in identifying aspects of occupational engagement and the influencing factors that generate occupationally focussed questions that are both individualistic and contextual. Such questions lead to concepts and theories of occupation that are embedded in occupational science. Furthermore, I have conceptualised occupation as a multi-faceted phenomenon that exists in the context of a domain and has particular forms. Its complex nature requires sensitive analysis as a prerequisite to analysing the components of occupational performance. The occupational domain and occupational form provide a context for understanding the meaning of occupation for individuals and consequently how issues such as occupational deprivation and injustice impact on occupational identity, balance, choice and control.

# References

Backman, C.L. (2010) Occupational balance and wellbeing. In: *Introduction to Occupation: The Art and Science of Living*, eds C.H. Christiansen and E.A. Townsend, 2nd edn, pp. 231–249. Upper Saddle River, NJ: Pearson.

Barber, M.D. (2006) Occupational science and the first-person perspective. *Journal of Occupational Science* 13(1), 94–96.

Brienes, E.B. (1995) *Occupational Therapy, Activities from Clay to Computers. Theory and Practice*. Philadelphia: F.A. Davis Company.

Christiansen, C. (1999) Defining lives: occupation as identity: an essay on competence, coherence, and the creation of meaning. *American Journal of Occupational Therapy* 53(6), 547–557.

Christiansen, C. (2004) Occupation and identity: Becoming who we are through what we do. In: *Introduction to Occupation: The Art and Science of Living*, eds C.H. Christiansen and E.A. Townsend, pp. 121–140. Upper Saddle River, NJ: Prentice Hall.

Clarke, F. (2006) One person's thoughts on the future of occupational science. *Journal of Occupational Science* 13(3), 167–179.

Csikszentmihalyi, M. (1996) *Creativity, Flow and the Psychology of Discovery and Invention*. New York: HarperCollins.

Dickie, V.A. (2003) The role of learning in quilt making. *Journal of Occupational Science* 10(3), 120–130.

Dickie, V.A., Cutchin, M.P. and Humphry, R. (2006) Occupation and transactional experience: a critique of individualism in occupational science. *Journal of Occupational Science* 13(1), 83–93.

French, G. (2002) Occupational disfranchisement in the dependency culture of a nursing home. *Journal of Occupational Science* 9(1), 28–37.

Glover, J. (2009) The literature of occupational science: a systematic, quantitative examination of peer-reviewed publications from 1996–2006. *Journal of Occupational Science* 16(2), 92–103.

Hagedorn, R. (1995) *Occupational Therapy Perspectives and Processes*. London: Churchill Livingstone.

Hagedorn, R. (1997) *Foundations for Practice in Occupational Therapy*. London: Churchill Livingstone.

Hocking, C. (2000a) Occupational science: a stock-take of accumulated insights. *Journal of Occupational Science* 7(2), 58–67.

Hocking, C. (2000b) Having and using objects in the Western world. *Journal of Occupational Science* 7(3), 148–157.

International Society for Occupational Science (ISOS) Interim executive (2007) *The Way Forward: Plan for ISOS*. http://www.isoccsci.org/ (accessed 3 May 2011).

Jakobsen, K. (2004) If work doesn't work: how to enable occupational justice. *Journal of Occupational Science* 11(3), 125–134.

Jarman, J. (2004) What is occupation? Interdisciplinary perspectives on defining and classifying human activity. In: *Introduction to Occupation: The Art and Science of Living*, eds C.H. Christiansen and E.A. Townsend), pp. 47–61. Upper Saddle River, NJ: Prentice Hall.

Laliberte-Rudman, D. (2002) Linking occupation and identity: lessons learned through qualitative exploration. *Journal of Occupational Science* 9(1), 12–19.

Mernar, T.J. (2006) Occupation, stress, and biomarkers: measuring the impact of occupational injustice. *Journal of Occupational Science* 13(3), 209–213.

Nagle, S., Valiant Cook, J. and Polatajko, H. (2002) Occupational choices of persons with severe and persistent mental illness. *Journal of Occupational Science* 9(2), 72–81.

Nelson, D. (1988) Occupation: form and performance. *American Journal of Occupational Therapy* 42(10), 633–641.

Nelson, D. (1994) Occupational form, occupational performance, and therapeutic occupation. In: *The Practice of the Future: Putting Occupation back into Therapy*, ed. C.B. Royeen. Rockville, MD: the American Occupational Therapy Association Inc.

Nelson, D. and Jepson-Thomas, J. (2003) Occupational form, occupational performance and a conceptual framework for therapeutic occupation. In: *Perspectives in Human Occupation Participation in Life*, eds P. Kramer, J. Hinojsa and C.B. Royeen, pp. 87–155. Philadelphia: Lippincott, Williams and Wilkins.

Pierce, D., Atler, K., Baltisberger, J., Hunter, E., Malkawi, S. and Parr, T. (2010) Occupational science: a data-based American perspective. *Journal of Occupational Science* 17(4), 204–215.

Reed, K.L. and Sanderson, S.N. (1999) *Concepts of Occupational Therapy*, 4th edn. Philadelphia: Lippincott, Williams and Wilkins.

Reynolds, F. (1997) Coping with chronic illness and disability through creative needlecraft. *British Journal of Occupational Therapy* 60(8), 352–356.

Riley, J. (2009) *Shaping textile-making as an occupational domain: Perspectives, contexts and meanings*. PhD thesis, Cardiff University.

Riley, J. (2011) Shaping textile-making: its occupational forms and domain. *Journal of Occupational Science* 18(4), 322–338.

Sennett, R. (2008) *The Craftsman*. London: Penguin Books.

Shils, E. (1981) *Tradition*. London: Faber & Faber.

Smith, D.L. and Hilton, C.L. (2008) An occupational justice perspective of domestic violence against women with disabilities. *Journal of Occupational Science* 15(3), 166–172.

Townsend, E., Stanton, S., Law, M., Polatajko, H., Baptiste, S., Thompson-Franson, T., Kramer, C., Swedlove, F., Brintnell, S. and Campanile, L. (2002) *Enabling Occupation: An Occupational Therapy Perspective*. Ottawa, ON: CAOT ACE.

Townsend, E. and Polatajko, H.J. (2007) *Enabling Occupation II: Advancing an Occupational Therapy Vision for Health, Well-being and Justice through Occupation*. Ottawa, ON: CAOT ACE.

Townsend, E. and Wilcock, A. (2004) Occupational justice. In: *Introduction to Occupation: The Art and Science of Living*, eds C.H. Christiansen and E.A. Townsend, pp. 243–268. Upper Saddle River, NJ: Prentice Hall.

Turpin, M. and Iwama, M.K. (2011) *Using Occupational Therapy Models in Practice, a Field Guide*. Edinburgh: Churchill Livingstone Elsevier.

University of Southern California (2009) *Occupational Science*. http://www.usc.edu/schools/ihp/ot/os/ (accessed 9 March 2009).

Wada, M., Backman, C.L. and Forwell, S.J. (2010) Theoretical perspectives of balance and the influence of gender ideologies. *Journal of Occupational Science* 17(2), 92–103.

Westhorp, P. (2003) Exploring balance as a concept in occupational science. *Journal of Occupational Science* 10(2), 99–106.

Whiteford, G. (2004) When people cannot participate: occupational deprivation. In: *Introduction to Occupation: The Art and Science of Living*, eds C.H. Christiansen and E.A. Townsend, pp. 221–242. Upper Saddle River, NJ: Prentice Hall.

Wilcock, A.A. (1993) A theory of the human need for occupation. *Journal of Occupational Science* 1(1), 17–24.

Wilcock, A.A. (1998) *An Occupational Perspective of Health*. Thorofare, NJ: Slack.

Wilcock, A.A. (1999) Reflections on doing, being and becoming. *Australian Occupational Therapy Journal* 46, 1–11.

Wilcock, A.A. (2006) *An Occupational Perspective of Health* 2nd edn. Thorofare, NJ: Slack.

Yerxa, E. (1998) Health and the human spirit of occupation. *American Journal of Occupational Therapy* 52(6), 412–418.

## Further reading

Christiansen C.H., and Townsend E.A. (eds) (2010) *Introduction to Occupation: The Art and Science of Living*, 2nd edn. Upper Saddle River, NJ: Pearson.

Glover, J. (2009) The literature of occupational science: A systematic, quantitative examination of peer-reviewed publications from 1996–2006. *Journal of Occupational Science* 16(2), 92–103.

Hocking, C. (2000) Occupational science: a stock-take of accumulated insights. *Journal of Occupational Science* 7(2), 58–67.

Kramer P., Hinojsa J. and Royeen, C.B. (eds) (2003) *Perspectives in Human Occupation Participation in Life*. Philadelphia: Lippincott, Williams and Wilkins.

# Chapter 15

# Myths around using theory in occupational therapy practice

*Alison Seymour, Gail Boniface and Louise Ingham*

---

**Key points**

- Practitioners and students often adhere to ideas around the use of theory in practice that do not necessarily have a basis in the theory
- These ideas can become facts over time, even though they are merely myths
- When ideas become myths they can restrict theory use if not challenged

---

## Introduction

In this, the final chapter, we acknowledge that there can still be strongly held ideas on the part of occupational therapists, educators and students related to embracing the use of theory within our profession. This is especially so when that theory is mainly viewed as having developed through custom and practice, as some of the comments we have heard whilst leading workshops on the use of occupational therapy professional models, such as 'but we've always done that', illustrate.

Using our own experiences and those of practitioner colleagues, we will now try to address some of the concerns and myths we often hear in respect to adopting theory; particularly those related to using occupational therapy professional models. We present these issues here either in the format of frequently asked questions or misconceptions (statements) about using occupational therapy professional models.

## Does using a model restrict my practice?

All of the occupational therapy conceptual models are based upon the philosophical underpinnings of the profession with the concepts of humanism, holism and occupations being central tenets. They are  not designed to dictate how practitioners should

---

*Using Occupational Therapy Theory in Practice*, First Edition. Edited by Gail Boniface and Alison Seymour.
© 2012 Blackwell Publishing Ltd. Published 2012 by Blackwell Publishing Ltd.

intervene, but rather to promote a professional focus and 'provide a conceptual structure by means of which clinical reasoning may take place' (Hagedorn 1995, p. 39). They are *models for* not *models of* practice (see Chapter 2). In other words, rather than restricting practice, a conceptual model challenges occupational therapists to more fully understand how individuals choose, experience and perform occupations and enables them to analyse the unique occupational difficulties each individual faces in daily life within their own environments. A model is not designed to be used in isolation from other evidence-based theory. In fact, Kielhofner (2008) postulated that the Model of Human Occupation (MOHO) 'was always intended to be used alongside other occupational therapy models and interdisciplinary concepts' (p. 4). He surmised that it is the use of models and approaches, in combination, that facilitates individually tailored and comprehensive occupational therapy practice. An understanding of conceptual models enables occupational therapists to either select from existing structures or to develop their own structures based upon the theoretical knowledge of the model. By this we mean that when using a particular occupational therapy professional model, there is *nothing to stop us using such things as assessments from another model or from a specific approach or devising our own tools based on the model.* What we might need to do in such an instance is to determine at what level we are assessing and choose our assessments accordingly. For example, we might be basing our practice within the sub-systems heterarchy of the MOHO, decide we need a very client-centred way of identifying the occupational performance issues our client has, identify that those issues are mostly psychologically based and probe further by using a more skills-based assessment from the cognitive behavioural approach's repertoire of assessments. Thus, we might initially use the Model of Human Occupation Screening Tool (MOHOST; Parkinson et al 2006) (see Chapter 12) to identify the client's issues within the separate occupational areas; the Canadian Occupational Performance Measure (COPM; Law et al 2005) (see Chapter 8 and 9) to help the client to set occupational goals and the Hospital Anxiety and Depression Scale (Zigmond and Snaith 1983) to ascertain the level of anxiety the client may present with. This could also be applicable in a physical way by, for example, using the concepts of the Canadian Model of Occupational Performance and Engagement (CMOP-E; Townsend and Polatajko 2007) as an initial assessment to identify the client's occupational performance issues, the Occupational Self-Assessment (Baron et al 2006) to set occupational goals and the Barthel index (Mahoney and Barthel 1965) to identify the client's specific self-care needs. Once we have assessed, of course, we will need to return to the occupational therapy model throughout the problem-solving process of planning, intervention and evaluation to ensure we stay true to the tenets of our profession. We should also remember that the use of models is a constantly developing process and, therefore, all occupational therapists have an opportunity to contribute to the development of professional conceptual models as they evolve, so one day our versions of assessments, plans and interventions based on our models could be put to more general use. After all, the refinement by us of our own occupational therapy professional models can lead to the development of our profession, not its restriction as long as we view our models as *models for* not *models of* practice (see Chapter 2).

## Will using a model be too time consuming when my service setting demands specific assessments?

Using specific assessments, for example those linked to a diagnosis, without first exploring how an individual needs to engage in their unique set of meaningful occupations, poses a significant risk of reductionism and failure to fully understand individuals as occupational beings. As we identified in the previous section, this does not negate the importance of such assessments for addressing the implications of a diagnosis on occupational interruption, but the use of a model-based assessment offers an effective starting point for client-centred occupational therapy practice.

Time *is* required to understand and document a service user's occupational strengths and the areas in which they have current occupational participation issues, both from their own frame of reference and also from the perspective of significant others. However, current policy drivers are demanding improved personalised outcomes. Taking the time needed to understand an occupational therapy conceptual model leads to a clearer establishment of the client-centred performance context, occupational, performance, and environmental issues and leads to overall outcomes being enhanced and ultimately costs are reduced (Neistadt 1995; Bowen 1996).

Previous chapters have shown that basing practice on an occupational therapy conceptual model enables practitioners to more effectively articulate their clinical reasoning and structure documentation more efficiently. Thus, although learning about the theory of the model may take time, it will enable practitioners to document observable and measurable baseline levels of occupational performance and focus on activities that hold true meaning and relevance for the service user. In turn, this helps facilitate effective recording of assessment and intervention that can be used for evaluating outcomes and developing evidence-based practice (Fisher 2009). Ultimately, investing time in this process is crucial to the practice of occupational therapy and to providing an evidence base that asserts the value of employing occupational therapists.

## Yes, but using a model duplicates documentation and conflicts with generic service frameworks, for example Unified/Single Assessment Process and the Care Programme Approach, 'how can I do both?'

It has already been identified that occupational therapy professional models offer flexible structures for organising and presenting occupational assessment data, whilst acknowledging that additional assessments may be needed to ensure a comprehensive baseline for planning and evaluation. It is widely accepted that assessment is the first step in the health care (and problem-solving) process and provides the foundation for effective intervention (Laver-Fawcett 2007). Many practice settings have specific initial assessment forms, some of which will already be based upon an occupational therapy professional model. However, in other service settings assessment documentation sits within generic service frameworks, such as the Unified/Single Assessment Process or the Care Programme Approach. Duplicating documentation onto different forms is not cost-effective and often it is possible to effectively record model-based occupational therapy assessment within generic forms by adding in appropriate *professionally* focused sub-headings or *profession-specific* additional assessments.

An illustration of this would be to use one of Kielhofner's basic approaches to organising documentation (Kielhofner 2008) when assessing occupational participation within the domains of a more generic assessment process. For example, when assessing washing, bathing or dressing within the activities of daily living domain, the assessment evidence could be examined and recorded by adding in the sub-headings of volitional issues, habituation, performance capacity, skills and environmental issues. Where local forms do not allow the space for this professional detail, attaching occupational therapy evidence sheets to the relevant domains may offer a way forward. Utilising an occupational therapy model will also ensure that occupational therapy is not merely limited, for example, to the domain of activities of daily living, as any occupational therapy model would require the practitioner to also consider productivity (work) and leisure as well as self-care (self-maintenance) or activities of daily living.

Where the requirement to use generic frameworks within the planning stages exists, similar principles may be applied. For example, the Care Programme Approach (CPA; Care Programme Approach Association 2011) presents generic care plan documentation; however, the headings on this form can be effectively applied to mapping out an occupational therapy plan. The addition of model-linked sub-headings such as productivity, leisure and self-care, can help clarify what needs to be addressed to reach the service user's desired occupational outcomes. Thus the occupational therapy plan may be a part of, or the entire, CPA care plan depending on the needs of the service user. Similarly, when using other generic or single assessment processes within organisations, the occupational therapist will need to complete the organisational paperwork. However, they will need to consider the nature of their professional assessments and plans within the generic format and use an occupational therapy model to structure the recording of those. This should then lead to the actions of the occupational therapist remaining occupational rather than performance skill based in nature.

## Are models compatible with care pathways?

The COT Strategy *Recovering Ordinary Lives* (COT 2006) challenges occupational therapists to build pathways of care that highlight what service users can expect from occupational therapy services; this includes mapping out the evidence base that underpins best practice, service user choices, timescales for service delivery and expected outcomes. Integrated Care Pathways (ICPs) are a means that determine multi-disciplinary, locally agreed practice guidelines for specific conditions and service users (Riley 1998). They are utilised as clinical governance tools and are not only expected to describe service processes within health and social care but also to include service standards with systems for monitoring and reviewing outcomes. Therefore, ICPs are also a tool for collating variances between planned and actual service delivery and identifying where service deficits exist. Although ICPs aim to increase the consistency of evidence-based services, pathways also need to accommodate the flexibility needed to meet individualised needs. To attempt to completely standardise occupational therapy practise for service user groups would impede the range of client-centred interventions that are developed from the use of an occupational therapy model. Earlier chapters of this book have established that occupational therapy conceptual models, and the range of assessments derived from them, offer a strong foundation both to the theoretical evidence base of the profession and to the occupational outcomes that we strive for collaboratively with service users. This evidence base should be acknowledged and included within local occupational therapy pathways and fed into the larger scale developments currently taking place, for example the work being undertaken by Local Health Communities to integrate clinical pathway areas within the *Map of Medicine* (NHS Institute for Innovation and Improvement 2009).

## Using the headings of a model as a *loosely based* checklist

Checking off headings from a model, without trying to understand and address a person's unique experience or more importantly understanding the theory that underpins the model, limits its use and detracts from the quality of the therapeutic relationship. It turns it into a *model of* rather than a *model for* (see Chapter 2) occupational therapy. It also results in failure to integrate the continued use of an occupational therapy professional model throughout the problem-solving process. Reed and Sanderson (1999) describe models as a guide for helping organise the practice of occupational therapy, but they also make the point that they are not recipes to dictate practice. Revisiting and reflecting on a model, for example to evaluate whether relevant aspects impacting on an individual's occupational functioning have been adequately considered, undoubtedly benefits practice and the confidence of developing practitioners. However, it is imperative to be responsive to the needs of service users in their own unique situations and changing environments. It is not realistic to expect a conceptual model to always have the answers. Thus, models will not always address an identified problem; when this situation is encountered, Reed and Sanderson (1999) suggest that the practitioner decides 'whether to revise the model, dispense with the model, or develop a new model' (p. 199). They warn practitioners about the limitations posed by overzealous model application and emphasise the need to review models to determine if other occupational therapy models might better guide current practice.

## Attempting to make the person fit the model

This is a similar pitfall to that described in the preceding text. The notion that *one size fits all* is not consistent with an ability to view each individual as unique. To be responsive practitioners, occupational therapists need to continually reflect on and adapt their practice. This not only necessitates careful consideration of how different models, assessments and approaches are utilised but also consideration of how interactions underpinned by theory are worded. For example, when using the questions suggested alongside a structured assessment like the Occupational Circumstances Assessment – Interview Rating Scale (OCAIRS; Forsyth et al 2005), it would be inappropriate to ask the questions in a rote manner without considering the specific needs of individuals and the individual circumstances within which the assessment is being carried out. Fisher (2009) cautions practitioners about asking questions using terms that have little meaning to service users, which could be experienced as threatening, or which are too broad/vague, for example when attempting to explore cultural issues or using terms like spirituality. In such instances, we would suggest that the occupational therapist should carefully consider *how* and indeed *whether* to use the terms that may be specific to an occupational therapy model. Altering Kielhofner's (2008) *volition* to *motivation*, for example, changes the meaning of the concept, whereas the Canadian Model's (Townsend et al 2002; Townsend and Polatajko 2007) use of the word spirituality portrays a concept that is either hard to grasp *or* only too easily interpreted as religiosity. The question the occupational therapist then has to ask themself is whether to use the word or alter the word to convey the model's concept to their client. Whichever decision is made, it is important that all of the occupational therapy model's concepts are considered to ensure holistic, occupationally based and client-centred occupational therapy.

## Confusing a model with a associated assessment

This most frequently occurs when an acronym for a model and a related assessment are similar. The obvious example of this is the CMOP-E (Townsend and Polatajko 2007) and the outcome measure linked to it, the COPM (Law et al 2005). Similarly, assessments linked to the MOHO, for example the MOHOST (Parkinson et al 2006) are occasionally confused for the parent model. It is important for occupational therapists to clearly differentiate the theoretical model from the subsequent assessments devised to help gather information relevant to the concepts of the parent model. Again, in our experience, practitioners often use associated assessments before they fully understand the theory which underpins its development. Therefore, we would strongly advocate that practitioners revisit the underpinning theoretical model before using associated assessments. Chapters 8 and 12 give practitioner accounts of the benefits to the individual and service in striving to understand the theory behind the occupational therapy model *before* rushing to use its assessments.

## Why doesn't a model give more guidance on intervention?

This is often asked in relation to the MOHO (Kielhofner 2008), probably because it is the most evidence-based model in relation to assessment and has the most associated assessments underpinned by the theory of the model. Interestingly Kielhofner is very clear about this issue. In the latest version of the model (Kielhofner 2008), when exploring performance capacity he acknowledges that approaches (although he refers to them as models) such as the bio mechanical approach, sensory integration and cognitive behavioural approaches are used by occupational therapists to understand and address specific performance capacity issues. What is important is how these approaches are used from an occupational therapy perspective, that is they should be used to develop individual, client-centred and occupationally focused interventions. This involves the process of professional thinking (Chapter 2) underpinned by the occupational therapy professional model, its associated assessments and knowledge of evidence-based approaches to intervention. Thus, an occupational therapy model that truly incorporates the theory and basic tenets of the profession should leave some room in its implementation for the therapist to utilise their professional thinking, otherwise it would become a directive *model of* the profession rather than a guiding *model for* the profession.

## Conclusion

In this concluding chapter, we have attempted to address some of the ideas, which over time, have become associated with the use of occupational therapy models and have gradually been turned into myths. The mythology has all been presented to us in some form or other by practitioners, students and academics. We have offered our views as to why these ideas are myths and attempted to challenge the mythology via our frequently asked questions. We would now wish to conclude by addressing the final myth that often surrounds and even envelopes occupational therapy models that one or other model is only appropriate or most appropriate for use in a specific particular setting. For example, we have heard it contended that Reed and Sanderson's (1999) model is only or mostly applicable in physical settings and that the MOHO (Kielhofner 2008) is most appropriate in a mental health setting. It is here that we must draw the reader's attention to the fact that the chapters wherein practitioners discuss their use of those two models (six and seven) do seem to give that impression, but this is only by chance and is *not a view that we hold!* We strongly believe (and recognise that others will disagree) that any occupational therapy model *can* and *should* be used in any setting as they all basically address very similar occupational, environmental and performance and engagement areas, which affect all of our clients, wherever they happen to receive our services.

## References

Baron, K., Kielhofner, G., Lyengar, A., Goldhammer, V. and Wolenski, J. (2006) *The Occupational Self Assessment (OSA) (version 2.2)*. Chicago: Model of Human Occupation Clearinghouse. Department of Occupational Therapy, College of Applied Health Sciences, University of Illinois at Chicago.

Bowen, R.E. (1996) The Issue is – should occupational therapy adopt a consumer-based model of service delivery? *American Journal of Occupational Therapy* 50, 899–902.

Care Programme Approach Association. http://cpaa.co.uk/thecareprogrammeapproach (accessed 23 May 2011).

College of Occupational Therapists (COT) (2006) *Recovering Ordinary Lives*. London: COT.

Fisher, A.G. (2009) *Occupational Therapy Intervention Process Model: A Model for Planning and Implementing Top-Down, Client-Centred, and Occupational-Based Interventions*. Fort Collins, CO: Three Star Press Inc.

Forsyth, K., Deshpande, S., Kielhofner, G., Henriksson, C., Haglund, L., Olson, L., Skinner, S. and Kulkarni, S. (2005) *The Occupational Circumstances Assessment – Interview and Rating Scale (OCAIRS) (version 4.0)*. Chicago: Model of Human Occupation Clearinghouse. University of Illinois at Chicago.

Hagedorn, R. (1995) *Occupational Therapy Perspectives and Processes*. Edinburgh: Churchill Livingstone.

Kielhofner, G. (2008) *Model of Human Occupation: Theory and Application*, 4th edn. Baltimore: Lippincott, Williams and Wilkins.

Laver-Fawcett, A.J. (2007) *Principles of Assessment and Outcome Measurement for Occupational Therapists and Physiotherapists: Theory, Skills and Application*. Oxford: John Wiley & Sons.

Law, M., Baptiste, S., Carswell, A., McColl, M., Polatajko, H. and Pollock, N. (2005) *Canadian Occupational Performance Measure*. Toronto: CAOT Publications.

Mahoney, F.I. and Barthel, D. (1965) Functional evaluation: The Barthel Index. *Maryland State Medical Journal* 14, 56–61.

Neistadt, M.E. (1995) Methods of assessing patients' priorities: A survey of adult physical dysfunction settings. *American Journal of Occupational Therapy* 49, 428–436.

NHS Institute for Innovation and Improvement. (2009) *Visualising and Integrating Clinical Pathways*. London: Map of Medicine Ltd.

Parkinson, S., Forsyth, K. and Kielhofner, G. (2006) *The Model of Human Occupation Screening Tool (version 2.0)*. Chicago: The Model of Human Occupation Clearinghouse. Department of Occupational Therapy, College of Applied Health Sciences, University of Illinois at Chicago.

Reed, L.R. and Sanderson, S.N. (1999) *Concepts of Occupational Therapy*, 4th edn. Philadelphia: Lippincott, Williams and Wilkins.

Riley, K. (1998) NPA Definition of a Pathway of Care. *National Pathways Association Newsletter*, Summer 1998.

Townsend, E., Stanton, S., Law, M., Polatajko, H., Baptiste, S., Thompson-Franson, T., Kramer, C., Swedlove, F., Brintnell, S. and Campanile, L. (2002) *Enabling Occupation: An Occupational Therapy Perspective*. Ottawa, ON: CAOT ACE.

Townsend, E.A. and Polatajko, H.J. (2007) *Enabling Occupation II: Advancing an Occupational Therapy Vision for Health, Well-being & Justice through Occupation*. Ottawa, ON: CAOT ACE.

Zigmond, A.S., and Snaith, R.P. (1983) The hospital anxiety and depression scale. *Acta Psychiatrica Scandinavica* 67, 361–370.

# Index

*Note*: Page numbers followed by italicised *f*'s and *b*'s indicate figures and boxes, respectively.

---

*Using Occupational Therapy Theory in Practice*, First Edition. Edited by Gail Boniface and Alison Seymour.
© 2012 Blackwell Publishing Ltd. Published 2012 by Blackwell Publishing Ltd.

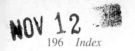